The FDA for Doctors

William H. Eaglstein

The FDA for Doctors

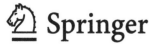 Springer

William H. Eaglstein, MD
Chairman Emeritus
Department of Dermatology
and Cutaneous Surgery
The University of Miami
Miller School of Medicine
Miami, FL
USA

ISBN 978-3-319-08361-2   ISBN 978-3-319-08362-9   (eBook)
DOI 10.1007/978-3-319-08362-9
Springer Cham Heidelberg New York Dordrecht London

Library of Congress Control Number: 2014946346

Printed on acid-free paper

Springer is part of Springer Science+Business Media (www.springer.com)

Preface

Because the title of this book is open to a number of interpretations, it is important to point out that this is not a "how-to" book. That is, the nitty gritty details of, for example, submitting an Investigative New Drugs exemption or initiating a New Drug Application are not a part of this book. Rather than offering guidance on the specifics of dealing with or interacting directly with FDA, this book is aimed at explaining, especially to doctors, FDA as an institution, understanding its nomenclature, its societal role, its policies, goals and challenges. Although almost all potential readers have some knowledge of FDA, few have an appreciation of the many specific areas of FDA authority. For example, how many realize that the USA is one of only two countries which allow direct-to-consumer drug advertising and that it is regulated by FDA? Or that FDA itself advertises to try to prevent young people from smoking cigarettes, and that all proprietary drug names must be approved by FDA?

This is not a book for those already deeply versed in FDA matters and I am not an FDA or regulatory expert, but rather a physician who, in addition to having had a fairly long career in academic medicine and a shorter second career in the pharmaceutical industry, has had a long-standing interest in FDA as well as the opportunity to be involved in FDA and FDA-related matters of many sorts.

In addition to having over 40 years of experience as a clinical investigator in many trials done for FDA registration, I have developed and worked on animal models which have and still serve to generate information which is used to identify and ultimately help garner approval for many drugs and devices. I have been a member of and ultimately chaired an FDA advisory committee, and have been a consultant to several divisions of the FDA. While serving as a Health Policy Fellow of the Robert Wood Johnson Foundation and the Institute of Medicine, I had the opportunity to serve on the US Senate Labor Committee, helping with its FDA oversight activities. Throughout my career, while in the University, as a consultant to companies and as an employee of companies, I have helped develop and execute projects and strategies aimed at securing FDA approvals, including presentations at meetings with FDA and to FDA advisory committees. I have written a number of articles and book chapters about FDA and FDA-related matters, taught medical students and residents about FDA and lectured to many post-graduate organizations on FDA matters, in addition to serving on their committees dealing with FDA matters. It is with this background and from a physician's perspective that I concluded that a book such as this would be of value and interest to physicians and possibly many others.

Prospective editors have asked me why physicians or others might be interested in this book and if reading it might make them better physicians. In my mind the information in this book will make physicians more thoughtful and insightful doctors. I believe it also has the potential to enrich their lives, linking them to the many broad social issues of which they are a part, although often unknowingly. Additionally, I hope that for some this book might be a launch pad for an interest or perhaps a medical hobby which will lead to important contributions, whether through a professional organization or more directly.

Finally, as is always the case, in the course of writing this book, I have probably learned far more than will many if not all of the ultimate readers. Importantly, although I have endeavored to avoid errors, misstatements and misrepresentations, I feel certain that there will be some points, hopefully subtle, with which people with deep expertise and specific knowledge of one or another element, will disagree or feel factual mistakes were made. Since this is a single author book they will have no trouble identifying the responsible party. I would welcome communications on such and apologize in advance for any errors as well.

San Francisco, CA, USA   William H. Eaglstein, MD

Acknowledgement

I am pleased to recognize the importance to this work of Dr. Harvey Blank who initially sparked my interest in FDA and FDA-related matters. Harvey was the Professor and Chairman of the Department of Dermatology at the University of Miami where I trained and spent most of my career in academic medicine. His having spent time in the pharmaceutical industry before becoming a full-time academic was one of the many reasons he had a special view of medicine.

I want to thank my longstanding colleague and friend, Patricia Mertz, who made it possible for me to participate in both clinical and laboratory research related to FDA registration over many years, even those during which administration often took me away from the front lines. Pat is a fantastic experimentalist who is always digging deeper into issues.

Professor David Taplin and Dr. Howard Maibach both played important early roles in my immersion into the world of clinical trials done for FDA approvals, and being a Fellow in the Robert Wood Johnson Health Policy Fellowship program afforded me important insights and perspective into the regulatory process at a policy level. Dr. Phillip Frost first gave me the opportunity to learn about and view the FDA from a perch inside the pharmaceutical industry. I thank them all and acknowledge their role in making me able to produce this work.

Most importantly I wish to thank my wife, Janet Eaglstein, who tolerated and encouraged me in writing this book and who served as an expert in-house editor. Her linguistic skills and quick mind are only matched by her ability with the comma!

Contents

Figure and Table Legends

Chapter 1
Doctors and the FDA

In medical school, students learn a tremendous volume of information. The topics they study are the basic or preclinical sciences such as anatomy, physiology, microbiology and pharmacology; the clinical sciences such as internal medicine, surgery, pediatrics, obstetrics and gynecology; and subspecialties such as cardiology and gastroenterology. These topics are studied by way of books, lectures, laboratory exercises, bedside observations and participation. However, the role of the Food and Drug Administration (FDA) in medicine is never a topic of intense study. It is perhaps mentioned in passing in pharmacology or discussed by clinical faculty on rounds. In fact, when I have asked them, many doctors and medical students have told me that FDA stands for Federal Drug Administration. Of course, the FDA does regulate drugs but it also regulates foods, cosmetics, supplements, biologics (for example, vaccines) and devices (for example, heart valves). Given FDA's broad regulatory powers in matters clearly related to health, how can physicians know and be taught so little about the FDA?

The answer is not so difficult to understand. First, officially, FDA has no role in regulating or controlling the practice of medicine. The regulation of the practice of medicine is a state, rather than federal matter. Each state has its own rules which are applied to the practice of medicine. Second, as regards what doctors may use in the practice of medicine, Congress and the courts have said that doctors can use any and all means in the practice of medicine which they (doctors) have a reasonable basis to believe might benefit patients. Hence, physicians need not concern themselves with knowledge of and about FDA since FDA cannot interfere with or dictate their practice of medicine. (While being able to treat with 'whatever means' seems reasonable, it presumes that doctors and their patients can actually get the 'means'. This may not be the case for agents not available because they are not approved for any indication or not otherwise generally available. Furthermore, Congress recently passed legislation which gives FDA the ability to restrict the doctors who can prescribe certain drugs.)

A third reason doctors pay little formal attention to FDA is that FDA's activities are so broad-reaching as to be unnoticeable to us in the course of every day practice

© Springer International Publishing Switzerland 2014
W.H. Eaglstein, *The FDA for Doctors*, DOI 10.1007/978-3-319-08362-9_1

in the same way we take little conscious notice of the hills, lakes or bridges, constituting the landscape in which we live our daily lives. That is to say that FDA actually creates much of the landscape in which doctors practice. And the FDA-determined landscape, just like the physical landscape, is accepted without reflection or much contemplation. As we rarely dwell on the inconvenience occasioned by the need to drive to a bridge in order to cross a river or to drive around a mountain, physicians take as a given that they only have certain drugs, devices and biologics at their disposal. New agents appear over time, just as over time new bridges shorten the route across the river. Thus FDA's activities are so influential they are actually rarely considered in the course of daily practice.

A fourth reason physicians know little about FDA is that although much of the core information upon which FDA makes decisions is based on scientific knowledge and practice activities, FDA's existential basis and its ability to act are derived from laws which reflect broad societal judgments. To the extent that FDA's existence and powers rest on legislative constructs rather than on science and clinically-based information, FDA is a topic easily out of the scope of medical training. To the extent that FDA's activities are reflective of social judgment, they reside more in the realm in which doctors, like all others, may or may not care to be active participants.

This book is based on the idea that many doctors would like to know more about FDA, in order to better understand many of the issues they feel are related to their practice, such as off-label drug usage, and also to enrich their professional lives and allow them to understand more deeply the many FDA related articles written in the popular press such as the New York Times and The Wall Street Journal. It is further based on the notion that doctors would prefer a somewhat formal way to learn about FDA, and on my personal bias that, after getting tuned-in to FDA (Agency) matters, doctors will be especially insightful about many of the issues surrounding FDA's activities. The Agency is a vast subject engaging thousands of lawyers, regulators, scientists, physicians, writers, legislators and many others directly and indirectly. This book aims to be an introductory overview written from a physician's perspective for physicians. It is organized along lines that emphasize issues which I believe would be most interesting to physicians. Much of it deals with nomenclature and definitions, since, as is true of all fields, one must understand the special concepts and vocabulary of the field.

In that regard, a special note about the word "approved" is appropriate early on. "Approved" in FDA parlance has several meanings. Principally it means "approved for introduction into interstate commerce or marketing" as in "an approved drug", that is, a drug approved for marketing in the United States. Other appropriate regulatory uses of the word "approved" will almost always be in connection with the drug's label, for example, an "approved use" or an "approved indication". These phrases refer to what use or conditions of use FDA has approved. Often, of course, physicians have found many uses or conditions of use, e.g., different dosages, which FDA has never considered and thus are not approved or placed on the label. To many if not most people, the word "approved" may carry a moral or judgmental connotation, which is not appropriate from a regulatory point of view. This judgmental connotation is often mistakenly the meaning understood by patients, especially when reading news articles condemning the "unapproved" use of certain agents by physicians. Even physicians are often unclear about so-called "unapproved" uses. Hence it is best to recognize that "unapproved" in the FDA context is a legal rather than a moral term. In fact, it would be best to use the phrase "off-label" whenever possible, such as an off-label indication or an off-label use.

Finally it is important to realize that much of FDA's regulatory power and role depend upon the federal government's powers over interstate commerce. Although this basis is obvious, the consequences of FDA being able to make us have or not have agents such as drugs and devices by approving or not approving their entrance into interstate commerce are so profound determining for example how we study and prove safety and efficacy, that we "lose track" of exactly what is the basis of FDA's powers.

Chapter 2
What Are Drugs?

FDA defines a drug in the following three ways: (1) articles intended for use in the diagnosis, cure, mitigation, treatment or prevention of disease in man or other animals; (2) articles (other than food) intended to affect the structure or any function of the body of man or other animals; and (3) articles recognized in the official United States Pharmacopeia, Homeopathic Pharmacopeia of the United States or National Formulary or any supplement to any of them (Table 2.1). FDA-approved drugs are classified as either non-prescription – so-called Over-the-Counter (OTC) drugs – or prescription drugs. The latter are mainly either New Drugs, including Biological Drugs (Biologics), or Generic Drugs. However, prescription drugs may also be in the Botanical or DESI (Drug Efficacy Study Implementation) category. FDA regulation of human drugs is by its Center for Drug Evaluation and Research (CDER) while veterinary drugs are regulated through its Center for Veterinary Medicine. By FDA definition all drugs, in contrast to devices (Table 2.2), work, that is, achieve their intended purpose by chemical action in or on the body or through being metabolized.

FDA's approval of a drug is actually an approval to market the drug by allowing it to be entered into interstate commerce. Although FDA does not offer patents (intellectual property) for drugs, it does grant marketing exclusivity, known simply as exclusivity. While patents which are granted by the Patent and Trademark Office are for 20 years, the duration of exclusivity, which is designed to strike a balance between new drug innovation and generics, or reward and encourage certain development activities, varies with the type of approval. For example, new chemical entity drugs are given 5 years of exclusivity and orphan drugs (those with a small potential market) are given 7 years of exclusivity.

© Springer International Publishing Switzerland 2014
W.H. Eaglstein, *The FDA for Doctors*, DOI 10.1007/978-3-319-08362-9_2

Table 2.1 FDA definitions of a drug

A drug is defined as:
Articles intended for use in the diagnosis, cure, mitigation, treatment, or prevention of disease in man or other animals.
Articles (other than food) intended to affect the structure or any function of the body of man or other animals.
Articles recognized in the official USP, HPUS or NF or any supplement to any of them.

Table 2.2 FDA definition of a device

A device
Intended to diagnose, cure, mitigate, treat, or prevent a disease or condition
or
Affect the function or structure of the body;
AND
Does not achieve its intended use through chemical action in /on body; and is not metabolized to achieve its purpose

Prescription Drugs, New Drugs and Drug Approval

A prescription drug is an approved drug or medication that requires a medical prescription in order to be obtained. Prescription drugs are consider to not be safe for use except under the supervision of a medical practitioner. They are also known as Rx for recipe or Rx-only drugs and as legend drugs, based on laws requiring that they carry a statement that they may only be sold by prescription. Prescription drugs stand in contrast to non-prescription or OTC drugs.

The words "new drug" can have a number of meanings. For example, when your patient starts taking a new medication it may be called a new drug. In addition, a drug which has recently come on the market may be called a new drug, while an agent being developed but not yet on the market is often also called a new drug. However, for the FDA a new drug is a drug for which the U.S. Food and Drug Administration requires premarketing approval. It is even possible for a new drug to have been on the market for many years. For example, an OTC product may have been on the market before an FDA OTC monograph on its drug ingredient was issued. Once the monograph is issued, the drug must either be approved by complying with the monograph or by submitting a New Drug Application. New drugs are approved based on information in a New Drug Application, or an NDA, and therefore new drugs are often called NDAs. In other contexts, primarily after they are on the market, new drugs are referred to as innovator drugs, brand name drugs, pioneers or originals.

The actual active agent in a drug is called the Active Pharmaceutical Ingredient (API). APIs that have never been marketed in the USA are referred to as New Molecular Entities (an earlier term for these APIs was New Chemical Entities).

Because drugs based on NMEs are considered to be most innovative and to offer the most medical progress, each year FDA publishes a list of approved NMEs. FDA calls the entire drug containing the API and other, usually inactive, ingredients, a drug product.

The process by which FDA approves new drugs is especially well worked out and broadly understood. Although not realized by most of the public and many physicians, the original law (1948) governing drugs in the US only required that drugs be safe. It was believed that physicians and patients would determine the effectiveness of drugs. From time to time, this idea – requiring only proof of safety before allowing a drug to be marketed, with the assumption that surely doctors and patients can determine efficacy and act accordingly – is suggested anew, especially as a method to speed the availability of new drugs. However, since 1962, to gain approval, drugs have had to be both safe and effective.

Since safety is always less than 100 %, FDA must weigh a drug's risks to its benefits, the so-called benefit-to-risk ratio, in making its final determination on marketing approval. Even when approved, the public and doctors should realize that this determination is made with the information available at the time. That is "at the time of approval" the known benefits outweighed the known risks. Of course, not only are drugs never 100 % safe, they are also never 100 % effective. FDA is inevitably criticized for its actions or inactions on both ends of this spectrum. When people believe excessive concerns about safety are preventing a new drug from being approved, FDA is at fault for people suffering or even dying because they cannot get a drug. Conversely, when a marketed drug is perceived to be too dangerous with too many side effects, FDA is at fault for allowing unsafe, dangerous drugs onto the market.

At present it is "agreed" that for NCEs, the process takes about 15 years and costs from $600 to $800 million. It should be noted that this cost is a composite sum including all of the costs of developing drugs that failed (the losers), the lost income that the invested money might have generated and many other non-obvious costs. In fact, many authorities contest this cost figure, pointing out that dividing the number of new drugs for a given year by all of the reported company R&D expenses for that year gives a much larger number, between 3.6 and 11 billion per new drug. Whatever the true cost, drug development is without any doubt an expensive and risky process. The ultimate regulatory goal of this costly process is submission by the sponsor of a new drug application (NDA) to FDA for marketing approval. For situations such as a new indication for an already approved drug, a change in dosage or dosing form, creation of a combination product where the active agents have already been approved and so forth, an intermediary approval pathway has been developed by FDA which allows companies to use the data FDA has already approved, in order to reduce the development costs. This process is known as the 505 (B) (2) pathway. It still requires a new drug approval application but attempts to avoid requiring the sponsor to duplicate work which was done for the original approval.

Some prescription drugs are known as Orphan Drugs. These are drugs or biologic products (drugs) which are indicated for diseases so rare that the market for them is thought to be quite limited. Orphan drug status was created in order to encourage the development of drugs for rare diseases, which by definition must affect less than 200,000 people. Sponsors whose drugs qualify are afforded certain opportunities such as tax credits for clinical development costs, a waiver of review fees and a period of marketing exclusivity. However, the orphan drug status designation does not alter the standard regulatory requirements and process for obtaining marketing approval. Safety and effectiveness of the orphan drug must be established through adequate and well-controlled human studies.

Biological Drugs

Sometimes referred to as Biologicals, Large Molecule Drugs or Biological Products, biological drugs constitute a special category of drugs whose API is a large, rather than small, molecule. They are regulated by FDA's Center for Biologics Evaluation and Research (CBER) and are described more fully in Chap. 4.

Generic Drugs

Biosimilars are not generics. By definition a generic drug is considered to be the same as a brand- name drug . It is to be comparable in dosage form, strength, route of administration, performance characteristics and intended use. Generics contain the same active ingredient (API) and have been tested to prove what is called "therapeutic equivalence" with the brand name or innovator drug. Usually the therapeutic equivalence determination is based on equivalent blood levels of the active ingredient or another so called "surrogate" or substitute end point. Thus, for example, a generic antibiotic produces blood levels equivalent to blood levels of the brand name antibiotic, but since its ability to treat infections has not been studied, the blood levels are substitute or surrogate end points. Surrogate endpoints are measures rather than clinical findings.

Most generic drugs are tested to document that the blood levels they produce are equivalent to the blood levels produced by the brand-named drug, which is also known as the reference listed drug. These blood studies are, of course, much less costly than clinical trials in which a disease is treated. Clinical trials are the single most costly part of the drug development process, costing at times hundreds of millions of dollars. Being able to do tests for blood levels rather than clinical trials is one of the main reasons the price of generic drugs is low. Having blood levels be the end point for FDA approval also ensures that generics will make it to the marketplace relatively quickly. In situations where no satisfactory surrogate end point exists, for example topical antibiotics for the treatment of impetigo, generic drugs are tested in clinical trials which are essentially the same as the trials needed for approval of a new drug.

However, most generic drugs can be approved based on blood levels, and since most of the safety and efficacy testing has already been done by the brand-name drug which is being referenced by the generic (hence the designation of reference listed drug), the application for a generic drug contains less information and is therefore called an Abbreviated New Drug Application or ANDA. Generic drugs are therefore sometimes called ANDAs just as new drugs are referred to as NDAs. Because generic drugs have only been tested to show therapeutic equivalent (mostly with blood tests), the label of the generic drug must be consistent with, essentially identical, to the label for the reference listed drug.

Recently the US Supreme Court found that manufacturers of generic drugs cannot be held responsible for claims based on failure of the label to warn of the generic drug's side effects. Both "failure to warn" and "design defect" claims were denied by the court decisions (PLIVA v. Mening 2011 and Mutual Pharmaceutical v. Bartlett 2012). This situation has meant that even when the manufacturers of generic drugs learn of side effects which are not on their drug's label they cannot apply for label changes. By contrast, manufacturers of the brand- name or reference labeled drug are responsible for changing their label in response to new information (Wyeth v. Levine 2009). Subsequently, one state court has even held that the company producing the brand-name product is liable for damages produced by the generic drug! This set of circumstances is an especially clear illustration of the so-called "law of unintended consequences". In response to this 'regulatory gap' between generic and brand-name product safety, FDA indicated it may allow generic manufacturers to independently change the safety section of their labels. However, this may be difficult because federal law mandates that generic manufacturers use the same labeling and drug design as the brand name. If generics were required to change their label independently it could drive up the price of generic drugs.

Non-prescription or Over-the-Counter (OTC) Drugs

Non-prescription drugs, often referred to as OTC drugs, are drugs which can be sold without a prescription. That is, they may be sold from a self-service shelf or over-the- counter rather than via a prescription order to the pharmacist. Non-prescription drugs generally have these characteristics: they are very very safe, the reason for their use can be determined by the lay person and they can be labeled in a way that allows the consumer to understand how to use them without the assistance of a physician or other learned intermediary.

OTC drugs can be marketed without a new drug application, if they comply with the so- called OTC monograph. Drugs that are marketed based on monograph compliance are occasionally referred to as monographed drugs. Of course, drugs approved by following the monograph are not eligible for New Drug Product

Exclusivity. The monographs are based on the active ingredients and they describe especially the active agent, the claims and labeling, which FDA recognizes will produce safe, effective and properly labeled OTC drugs. Drugs intended for OTC distribution, for which there is no monograph, may be approved by the NDA process used for other new drugs. This pathway may require so-called label comprehension and/or use studies to document that the lay person can self-diagnose, understand and follow the label in self-treating.

On occasion, sponsors or the public petition FDA to switch a drug's status from prescription to OTC. FDA's determination will be based, as noted, on the drug's safety, the ability of the public to recognize when to use the drug and understand how to use it safely. To help ensure the safety of these OTC switches, as they are called, FDA will usually require a dose reduction (often a 50 % reduction) so that the OTC drug will contain a lower dose of the active agent than the prescription drug. Generally both the prescription and the OTC agent will remain available on the market. About 30 % of currently marketed OTC drugs are products that have been switched from prescription to OTC.

Some non-prescription drugs are now not allowed to be sold over the counter even though a prescription is not required for their purchase. Examples include drugs containing pseudoephedrine and drugs for emergency birth control. To buy these non-prescription drugs the purchaser must ask for and be given the agent and may, for example in the case of pseudoephedrine, be required to sign a register designed to keep track of and prevent excessive purchases thought to be associated with illicit drug production. Some US states have laws governing the sale of OTC drugs which might require that a sale be made only after a pharmacist has educated the buyer or confirmed the person's need.

Because OTC drugs offer many benefits, including quick access and reduced costs, FDA is often encouraged to explore methods of expanding their availability and use. Ideas proposed include greater utilization of pharmacists for on-site education and screening to allow a broader range of OTC agents, and high-tech pharmacy kiosks or websites utilizing algorithms to determine the appropriate OTC agent. Physicians have been concerned about issues such as OTC treatment for chronic conditions, which can change their morbidity over time, and the potentially dangerous mixing and matching of more potent OTC agents should they be approved.

Drug Efficacy Study Implementation (DESI) Drugs

"DESI" drugs are drugs which were approved between 1938 and 1962, a period when approval was based only on a drug's safety. In that era efficacy determination was left to the manufacturers, scientists, doctors and patients, without supervision and approval by FDA. In 1962, in response to the Thalidomide debacle in Europe (the FDA never approved Thalidomide because of safety concerns), Congress passed the Kefauver Amendments to the FDC act which, among other things, required that in addition to being safe, candidate drugs must prove they work in order to be approved for marketing. The Kefauver Amendments also required that FDA evaluate all of the already marketed drugs and confirm or ensure that they were also effective.

To evaluate the efficacy of all of the drugs approved and marketed before 1962, FDA developed a process called the Drug Efficacy Study Implementation, hence the name DESI. This was a large undertaking which because of limited resources, FDA contracted to the National Academy of Sciences/National Research Council and in which may doctors throughout the country participated on an essentially volunteer basis. The available studies and literature on more than 3,000 products and over 16,000 therapeutic claims were evaluated. By 1984, conclusions and rulings on 3,443 products were completed. Most of the pre-1962 drugs, 2,225, were ruled to be effective and remained on the market. Others were either withdrawn or went through a new but abbreviated approval process. However, the FDA determination of efficacy of some of the drugs approved before 1962 (and some drugs which are similar or related) has not been concluded and their status is considered by the Agency to be pending. These drugs are referred to as DESI drugs and they continue to be marketed. Examples of commonly used DESI drugs include colchicine and phenobarbital. DESI drugs are therefore marketed without approval and they are at risk of an FDA determination that they are not effective. Additionally, should a sponsor gain approval for a DESI drug by way of an NDA, companies marketing the same DESI drug would be required to withdraw their product. Finally, there are a few drugs which were never considered in the DESI process and which are still marketed. Some people have referred to these as DESI 2 drugs in order to suggest that they would be included in a second DESI process should there ever be one.

Both doctors and the public might be surprised to know that FDA is on record as indicating concern that these drugs, which are marketed "illegally", might not meet current standards of safety and efficacy and might not be properly labeled, posing a serious public health concern. This is especially the case when one realizes that hundreds of such drugs are still marketed in the United States. In addition to the concerns related above, DESI and other unapproved but marketed drugs are at risk of being declared less than effective and ineligible for reimbursement by federal, state and private health plans.

Botanical Drugs

There are many botanical products on the market in the United States. Depending on its labeling and intended use, a botanical product can be a food, a dietary supplement or a drug. Botanical products consumed primarily for their taste, aroma, or nutritive value are regulated as foods. Botanical products which are dietary supplements are also not regulated as drugs.

Although the pathways for approval of botanical drugs have been developed for some time, as of the middle of 2013, there were only two FDA-approved botanical drugs. The first was a tea-derived topical ointment to treat warts, while the second, approved 8 years after the first, is a tree sap derived oral anti-diarrheal for HIV patients.

As is the case for all drugs, botanical drugs are intended to treat, diagnose, mitigate or prevent a disease. Unlike most other drugs, however, botanical drugs are complex mixtures which lack a distinct or known active pharmaceutical ingredient (API), and, importantly, there must be evidence of substantial and safe human use prior to their approval. Botanical drug products consist of vegetable materials, which may include algae and macroscopic fungi. Highly purified or modified botanically-derived substances are not considered botanical drugs. A botanical drug product may be available as a solution, powder, tablet, capsule, elixir, topical or injection.

Although their active ingredient(s) need not be known, botanical drugs are required to have validated processes to ensure that their manufacture is consistent from batch to batch. As plant-derived products they might have a variety of active ingredients but are not subject to regulations applicable to combination drug products. As noted, the development of botanical drugs will allow consideration of their having been safely used for long periods of time by many people in the US or elsewhere. As such, the safety requirements for initial studies will be lower than those for NCEs.

For doctors, whether a drug is a botanical or as is more common, a synthesized small molecule, is of no great import if it can be therapeutically useful for a given patient. However, contemporary patients are frequently more receptive to the idea of plant-derived agents and as such more botanical drugs might be welcomed. When the FDA's Guidance on Botanical Drugs was issued in 2004, many anticipated it would stimulate a helpful and profitable synthesis of the body of empiric knowledge in the herbal medicine area with some of the rigor of Western medicine and result in a flood of new products. This hope has as yet not been realized despite the projected large markets and public enthusiasm for such.

Me-Too Drugs

Me-too drugs are not a regulatory drug category and not a category or term used by FDA. However, many people criticize FDA for approving me-too drugs and propose that FDA should have a different regulatory standard for them. The me-too drug designation is used in a number of ways, even by some to mean a generic drug. Its historic and most accurate use is to describe a drug with a mechanism of action similar to a drug already on the market. Although chemically distinct, the me-too drug will often have a chemical structure that is very much like the drug that created the therapeutic category – the so called first-to-market drug. These category-creating drugs are also called innovator or breakthrough drugs. Corticosteroids, antihistamines and statins are familiar examples.

Critics of me-too drugs have asserted they represent a poor allocation of resources. The critics believe that drug developers find it easier to slightly modify existing drugs and get them approved as new drugs which are sold at high prices than to try to develop really new drugs. The assertion is that this is a wasteful, mis-application of resources in a very resource-intensive circumstance. As a remedy, some want FDA to refuse to approve me-too drugs which are not superior to the category-creating drug.

Critics of me-too drugs suggest that after a breakthrough drug is produced, another company can create a modified version of the drug based on the prior work creating the break-through agent. However, the development of many me-too drugs was undertaken in the same time frame as the breakthrough drug and was usually based on identical basic science insights. As such, drugs that reach the market fairly quickly after the breakthrough drug, sometimes called follow-on drugs, were not breakthrough drugs only because they lost the race to the market. Other reasons doctors in particular might favor the availability of me-too drugs are that often the first drug to market proves later to have an unacceptable and unrecognized toxicity or is simply less effective than the me-too drug, or patients often fail to respond to one of the class but do respond to another, and frequently other indications or uses are found for one of the me-too drugs after approval. As regards the idea that because companies use all of their resources developing me-too drugs and thereby fail to develop more innovative drugs, FDA's study comparing the number of approvals of innovative drugs and advance-in-class me-too drugs, which they classify as addition-to-class drugs, does not support the idea that there is an innovation gap or crisis.

Chapter 3
What Are Devices?

Devices are similar to drugs, being articles (instruments, apparatus, implements, contrivances or implants) that are intended to diagnose, cure, mitigate, treat or prevent a disease or condition, or articles that affect the structure or function of the body. Devices are regulated by the Center for Devices and Radiological Health (CDRH). The difference between drugs and devices is that devices do not achieve their "intended use" through chemical action in or on the body or through being metabolized (Table 2.2). Most doctors have not been taught about this fairly clear distinction between a drug, which acts chemically, and a device, which does not produce its effects chemically. Because there have recently been so many combinations of a drug and a device, for example, coronary artery stents containing drugs which may prevent occlusive new tissue growths, combination categories have been recognized. "Combination Drug" indicates that the primary mechanism-of-action is as a drug, in which case the combination will have to go through the drug approval process and be regulated as a drug. "Combination Device" indicates that the primary action is as a device, with the regulatory pathway being as a device. (Combination Agents Chap. 5).

Broadly, whether an article is a drug or a device is not of great moment to doctors since we are more concerned with the specifics of a patient's circumstances and how the article will help the patient. We are very interested in detailed information about the article and are not concerned about its regulatory classification by FDA. However, the FDA classification has many implications for doctors and patients, especially as regards how easily an article becomes marketed and hence available for doctors to use.

The type of approval will also be important in determining what is allowed on the product's label. The FDA requirements for approving drugs are considerably higher, more costly and time consuming than they are for most devices. For example, while a device might easily reach the market in 1–2 years, drugs will usually require from 7 to 15 years or more, depending upon the drug's novelty. Also, once a new device is allowed on the market by FDA, one or several similar devices will usually reach the marketplace within 2 years. The marketing of these similar devices almost always results in a significant price reduction of the original and the subsequent

© Springer International Publishing Switzerland 2014
W.H. Eaglstein, *The FDA for Doctors*, DOI 10.1007/978-3-319-08362-9_3

Table 3.1 Device class
examples

Device classes
Class I – tongue depressor, gauze
Class II – 98 %, 510k
Lasers, ultrasound, sutures
Class III – full premarket review
Fillers, cellular dressings
98 % of devices are class II and many use the 510k route

agents. For novel drugs (New Chemical Entities) or biological drugs, a similar product is likely to take many years to be approved while a generic version must await the end of patent protection and any FDA provided marketing exclusivity time.

An article's classification as a drug or device also determines how much might be known about an article's functions and how it is labeled and promoted. In almost all cases, much less will be known about devices, although, as discussed below, doctors will be told about many unique properties of the newest devices. Interestingly, there is also a great difference in how devices can be promoted to doctors. For example, although not illegal, the FDA processes for allowing companies to give samples to doctors are so demanding that the era of simply handing out samples to doctors at medical meetings and elsewhere has ended. By contrast, certain devices, supplements and cosmetics are readily available to doctors at medical meetings and elsewhere.

For regulatory purposes devices are divided into classes I, II and III, from least to most regulated (Table 3.1). Most devices, about 98 %, are Class II. They are approved via an application known as a 510(k), after the regulation describing these types of submissions. When reading about class II devices and the 510(k) application one encounters phrases such as 510(k) route, 510(k) reviews, 510(k) submissions, 510(k) clearances and 510(k) approvals. The unique and very important feature of the 510(k) application is that the device for which approval is sought by the 510(k) route, only needs to be "substantially equivalent" to a device already marketed. The already-marketed device is called the "predicate device". Substantial equivalence implies that the new device is similar in design, material, chemical composition, energy source, manufacturing process, intended use, function, safety and effectiveness to the predicate device rather than identical to it. If cleared by FDA, the new device's labeled claims will be the same as that of the predicate. In about 90 % of the approximately 5,000 annual 510(k) applications, no new clinical research data is required or submitted in order to obtain 510k approval. This stands in great contrast to the requirements for most new drugs and biologics and obviates the tremendous costs of generating clinical proof of safety and efficacy (NCEs/new drugs) or bioequivalence (generics).

The 510(k) application is unique. There is not an analogue or similar approval mechanism for drugs or biologics. Because this approval mechanism is relatively rapid and inexpensive, sponsors often try to have articles approved by the 510(k) process. This approval process has given rise to what has been called "the 510(k) paradox" referring to the frequently encountered situation whereby a device is "cleared" (FDA clears rather than approves devices) because it is judged by FDA to be substantially equivalent to a predicate device, yet when doctors and the public hear about it, the recently cleared device is being promoted as an innovative, advanced product. Examples of this abound in the many lasers on the market almost all of which are approved because they are substantially equivalent to a laser already on the market, yet many are marketed as new breakthrough devices able to do what no other device can do. Class II devices are also required to meet and follow general requirements and special requirements based on the type of device. Such requirements are spelled out in FDA guidelines and include requirements such as meeting performance standards and keeping patient registries.

The least stringently regulated device category, Class I, is the lowest regulatory level. Examples of Class I devices are gauze, scalpels and tongue depressors. They are often exempt, meaning that they are on an FDA list of devices which can be marketed simply by meeting the general controls such as following Good Manufacturing Practices, ensuring labeling quality systems and records.

Class III devices are those which support or sustain life, or are of substantial importance in preventing impairment of health, or which present a potential, unreasonable risk of illness or injury. For example, devices such as heart valves, implanted stimulators and image analyzers are important in supporting life and preventing impairment of health, while devices such as breast implants and injectable fillers, which have considerable risk of producing illness or injury, are all in Class III. Class III devices require a pre-market approval application (PMA). The PMA is the device analogue of the drug New Drug Application (NDA) which, as mentioned, requires studies costing millions of dollars and taking many years. The PMA process requires clinical trials done under FDA approval (known as an Investigational Device Exemption) allowing the use of an investigational device. The studies must document the safety and effectiveness, adverse reactions and complications, device failures and replacements, patient information, patient complaints, tabulations of data from all individual subjects, results of statistical analyses, and any other information from the clinical investigations. Despite these more demanding requirements, the PMA requirements are still generally much less rigorous than the New Drug Application requirements. For example, while a drug approval requires two large randomized controlled trials, a PMA would usually only require one such trial. In addition, the review time and review cost of the PMA is less than that of the NDA. For example, the review fees for a new drug are over $1 million while for devices the fee is below $400,000.

Class III devices are also held to controls over manufacturing and performance and patient registries. Compared to drugs, devices are generally far less costly to develop, and while there are many more devices developed over any given time period, the market-life of devices, or at least the time when they are without substantial competition, is often only several years, compared to drugs which frequently have market-lives and periods of exclusivity of many decades.

As with most regulatory matters there are methodologies and pathways designed for special circumstances. Worthy of note in the device area is the Humanitarian Device Exemption pathway. So called Humanitarian Use Devices may be cleared by this pathway if they meet the requirements of a PMA submission but importantly for the Humanitarian Device Exemption approval, the PMA need not have clinical trial evidence of the device's efficacy. This humanitarian pathway is only available in situations in which the disease or circumstance (often this is a subgroup or sub-circumstance of a disease rather than all of those with the disease itself) to be treated or diagnosed by the device affects less than 4,000 people per year in the United States. Although the applicant is not required to have clinical investigations proving the device is effective, there must be evidence that the device is not unreasonably dangerous and that its probable benefit outweighs its possible risks. Furthermore, the applicant must document that there is not another device to do the job and that the applicant could not bring the device to the market without the exemption.

In summary, devices are agents which produce their effect physically rather than chemically. For physicians and others involved in making decisions regarding diagnosis and therapy, it is important to understand the often limited meaning of the claim that a device has been approved by FDA. In fact, to limit the impact of its approval, FDA only uses the word "cleared" to describe its marketing permission for devices. Physicians should also be aware that the amount of clinical information and level of evidence supporting the efficacy and safety of devices is not at all up to the standard physicians are accustomed to when they are considering the use of drugs.

Finally, a note about devices and surgery. Clearly, devices, scalpels, sutures, sponges are critical to doing surgery, and often the aim of the surgery is, in large measure, to implant a device into the body. However, although the devices are subject to FDA regulatory requirements and review, which can be intense or superficial depending on the device category, surgery itself is not regulated by FDA. Put another way, should you as a surgeon have a new method of doing your procedure there is no regulatory body to require determination that the new technique is safe or effective. Of course, hospitals and states do afford a level of oversight but this at best is only sufficient to avoid extremely unsafe circumstances. It would clearly be insufficient to evaluate more subtle variations between the new surgical procedure and the standard surgical approach.

Chapter 4
What Are Biologics, Biological Products and Biological Drugs?

Following the deaths of 14 children from contaminated antitoxins and smallpox vaccines, Congress in 1902 passed the Biologics Control Act, which is also known as The Virus-Toxin Law. This act required manufacturers to be licensed for safety and was a precursor and model for the Food Drugs and Cosmetics Act of 1938 which also emphasized safety. Most biologics or biological products fit the FDA definition of a drug and may be called biological drugs. They are medical products made from living organisms or derived from natural sources which may be animal, human or micro organismal. They can be composed of sugars, proteins or nucleic acids, or a combination of these substances. Biologicals may also be living entities, such as cells and tissues for use as cell or tissue therapy. They are often produced by biotechnology methods.

The Product License Application, which is similar to a New Drug Application, emphasizes that the manufacturing facilities obtain approval of their ability to produce products that are "safe, pure and potent". Of course, all drug manufacturers must produce safe, pure and potent products. However, the rigor needed to do so with biological drugs is such that the regulations pay special attention to the manufacturing process. Although, broadly, biologics or biological drugs are medical products made with living organisms, the technical definition in the US Code of Federal Regulations written in 1902 defines a biologic product as "any virus, therapeutic serum, antitoxin or analogous product applicable to the prevention, treatment or cure of diseases or injuries of man." In medical circles today, the word "biologics" usually refers to a subset of drugs which are distinguished by their manufacturing process or sourcing. Many of the therapeutic biologics used in medicine today are primarily regulated by FDA's Center for Drug Evaluation and Research with consultation, rather than primary responsibility, from the Center for Biologics Evaluation and Research. In addition to having a different regulatory history than other drugs (at one time NIH regulated biologics), biologics differ from other drugs in ways which make understandable their being regulated somewhat

© Springer International Publishing Switzerland 2014
W.H. Eaglstein, *The FDA for Doctors*, DOI 10.1007/978-3-319-08362-9_4

differently than small molecule drugs. Among the important differences between drugs which can be produced by chemical synthesis and biological drugs are that biologics:

1. Are only produced by living systems (but are not simply metabolites);
2. Have large molecular weights and high structural complexity (many of the contemporary biologics are large proteins);
3. Are inherently heterogeneous in the molecular species present;
4. Have an impurities profile dependent upon the processes used to make each batch;
5. Have activity which is very sensitive to physical conditions, e.g., temperature and shear forces, and enzymatic activity; and
6. Usually require bioassays for batch release and stability assessment rather than chemical tests.

Some of the more obvious clinical implications of these features include that biologics differ in effects depending on the manufacturing techniques; they might transmit an infectious agent; and, often being proteins which will denature with heat, they need to be kept refrigerated prior to use. This concern also imposes the burden on travelers to carry their medication in cool conditions. Until recently it had been FDA's position that there could be no "generic biologics" because the inherent structural complexity, heterogeneity and manufacturing process did not lend themselves to being copied exactly. However, FDA has recently issued Guidances and policies indicating that it will be possible to recognize what in Europe have been called biosimilars or "follow-on biologics". They are versions of the pioneer or original biologics which, while not exact molecular copies of the innovator biologic, have the same mechanism of action and clinical effects as the original biologic. They resemble the innovator in the same way as the drugs in families such as the statins or H2 blockers are in the same category but are not molecularly the same. However, unlike drugs in the same family, they are presently required to have the exact clinical effects. Biosimilars are to be approved by way of a full NDA or Biologic License Application (BLA). To be substituted for the innovator biologic, biosimilars are to be deemed "interchangeable" by FDA in a process which is separate from the initial approval process. Hence, in the biologics area there is as yet no way to develop inexpensive generic agents as we know them in the traditional drug category. That is, the pathway whereby rather inexpensive testing, such as showing that a generic drug has blood levels comparable to the innovator drug constitutes evidence of therapeutic equivalence sufficient for approval, is not available for biosimilars. Obviously the regulation of biologic products is demanding and complex. Of course for doctors the key is not how an agent is regulated but that it is manufactured and tested properly and will safely produce the desired effects.

Chapter 5
What Are Combination Products?

Combination products are made of agents in different regulatory categories. The number of such products is growing rapidly (about 8 %/year) with a market estimated at between $75 and $100 million yearly. The common categories are: drug eluting stents, infusion pumps, bone graft implants, photodynamic therapy, wound care combination devices, inhalers and transdermal patches.

Once combinations of agents in different regulatory categories became common, for example, a coronary artery stent device which contains and releases a drug which may prevent occlusive new tissue growths, so called combination product categories were defined by FDA. I imagine that to doctors it will be surprising how complex such a seemingly simple category can actually be. The categories include:

1. Products comprised of two or more regulated components (i.e., drug/device, biologic/device, drug/biologic, or drug/device/biologic) that are physically, chemically, or otherwise combined or mixed and produced as a single entity; for example, a monoclonal antibody (biologic) combined with a chemotherapeutic drug;
2. Two or more separate products packaged together in a single package or as a unit and composed of drug and device products, device and biological products, or biological and drug products, such as a surgical tray containing lidocaine (drug) and syringes and scalpels (devices);
3. A drug, device, or biological product packaged separately that according to its purposed labeling is intended for use only with an approved individually specified drug, device, or biological product, where both are required to achieve the intended use, indication, or effect, and where, upon approval of the proposed product, the labeling of the approved product would need to be changed (e.g., to reflect a change in intended use, dosage form, strength, route of administration, or significant change in dose), such as a photosensitizing drug and a laser device;
4. Any investigational drug, device, or biological product packaged separately that according to its proposed labeling is for use only with another individually specified investigational drug, device, or biological product, where both are required to achieve the intended use, indication, or effect. A drug containing two or more

© Springer International Publishing Switzerland 2014
W.H. Eaglstein, *The FDA for Doctors*, DOI 10.1007/978-3-319-08362-9_5

actives is not a combination product but remains a drug. Similarly, combinations of two or more biologicals or two or more devices would not be combination products. Combinations of a drug, device or biological with other regulated agents such as a cosmetic or a nutritional supplement would not be combination products.

Combination products are among the most cutting edge products in medicine. By bringing together products which would each be regulated by a different Center in FDA, each with different regulatory requirements, combination products create challenging policy, regulatory, review and management issues. For example, the different approval pathways between the combination product components need to be synthesized. In doing so, the requirements for most elements of approval from preclinical to clinical and manufacturing to promotion will be affected. Even combinations of already approved products, such as an approved device and an approved drug, when used in combination may result in needs and adverse events not seen with either alone.

In order to help clarify and to adjudicate such issues, the Congress and FDA have created the Office of Combination Products (OCP). The primary duties of OCP are to designate one of the FDA Centers (Drugs, Biologics or Devices) with primary responsibility for the combination product. While the Center, not OCP, is responsible for the scientific or technical review, OCP is responsible for ensuring that the premarket review is done in a timely fashion, which may require coordinating work between the Centers, and ensuring post-marketing review of combination products again by the Centers. In assigning jurisdiction and lead responsibility for a product to one of the Centers, the OCP is guided by its determination of the product's primary mode of action, which FDA defines as "the single mode of action of a combination product that provides the most important therapeutic action of the combination product." Hence, if the biologic is the primary mode of action of a combination device-biologic, the Center for Biologics would be assigned primary responsibility for the combination. If the single most important mechanism of action cannot be determined, FDA guidelines lead to assigning based on the assignment of similar products or to the Center with the most experience with such products. The pathway for approval would be that of the assigned Center although the regulations for manufacture of each component would that of the relevant Center.

Although for convenience, phrases such as "Combination Product Drug" or "Combination Drug" are often used to indicate a combination product whose primary mechanism-of-action is as a drug, such phrases might lead to confusion with what is known as a fixed dose drug combination or fixed dose combination, known also as FDC, which is a drug containing two or more active agents in fixed proportions. These are usually pills such as the combination retrovirals available to treat AIDS. These so called FDCs are also referred to as combination drugs or even combination drug products. For clarity the phrase combination device drug should probably be used, however it is a bit awkward for facile communication. Regardless of which terminology is used the idea is to convey by using drug as the final word that the combination product is considered by FDA to have a drug activity as its primary action and that it will be approved and regulated primarily by the drug center. Similarly, "Combination Device", combination drug device or combination product device indicates that the primary action is as a device, with the primary regulatory group being the device group. Although sponsors may recommend to FDA how or by which Center of FDA their proposed combination product should be regulated, the ultimate determination as to which group has primary regulatory jurisdiction is made by the OCP. Most often the primary Center consults and or collaborates with the other relevant Center(s) in reaching its determinations for pre-market approval and other matters.

Chapter 6
What Are Dietary Supplements and Nutraceuticals?

In the US, dietary supplement annual sales are about $30 billion annually, which is in the same sales range of several of the large pharmaceutical, or so called Big Pharma, companies. As doctors, we know how often people take one or more supplements with the idea that they are having a medicinal effect. A dietary supplement is a product that contains nutrients derived from food products that are concentrated in liquid or capsule form. Strictly speaking, dietary supplements, or simply supplements, are a subcategory of foods, not drugs. In 1994 Congress defined the term "dietary supplement" as a product taken by mouth that contains a "dietary ingredient" intended to supplement the diet. By law a dietary ingredient must be one or a combination of compounds specified in the Dietary and Health Education Act, such as vitamins, minerals, herbs or other botanicals and amino acids.

In the name of deregulation, the Dietary Supplement Health and Education Act of 1994 (DSHEA) restricted the FDA from exerting drug regulatory authority over dietary supplements as long as manufacturers made no claims about preventing or treating disease. As a result, the FDA currently regulates dietary supplements as a category of food but under the special provisions of the Dietary Supplement Health and Education Act, and not as drugs. In addition, the 1994 legislation requires that to remove a supplement from the market because of safety issues, the FDA must demonstrate that individual supplements are unsafe using its adverse events reporting system, which may capture only 1–10 % of all adverse events linked to supplements. According to the Act, the companies selling supplements are responsible for determining that their products are safe, and for determining that there is adequate evidence to substantiate structure and function claims about the supplements. Although not a term recognized by FDA, some supplements are known by doctors and the public as "nutraceuticals" in order to convey the idea that they are nutrients with pharmaceutical properties or activities. A similar term, cosmeceuticals, is applied to topical agents while nutraceuticals refers only to orally administered agents. The idea of supplements (dietary nutrients) having

© Springer International Publishing Switzerland 2014
W.H. Eaglstein, *The FDA for Doctors*, DOI 10.1007/978-3-319-08362-9_6

pharmaceutical properties is fortified by the legal provision contained in the DSHEA that so called "structure and function" claims can be made for supplements.

Congress passed the DSHEA allowing structure/function claims in response to public pressure to allow supplement labeling, which would give the average consumer information and guidance about nutrients or dietary ingredients for which there was basic science but not clinical science evidence suggesting a desirable "health outcome". Structure/function claims allow description of the effect of a dietary ingredient in maintaining normal structure and function in humans. FDA-provided examples of structure and function claims are: "calcium builds strong bones" or "fiber maintains bowel regularity". However, as the public and physicians know, many labeled claims go well beyond the constrained claims. For example, a seaweed extract label reads "Use as a dietary sea vegetable supplement for natural detoxification, weight management or immune support." Is detoxification treatment of a medical disease or state? What is weight management? And while supporting the immune system most closely adheres to the legal idea of maintaining structure and function, doctors would wonder how the immune system is supported and how would the public know when their immune system needs help with its support. In any given person is the immune system supported in its endeavor to help overcome an infection or fight incipient cancer, or is it supported in causing an immune-mediated disease such as rheumatoid arthritis? Some supplements have almost no indication of use with one combination of disparate ingredients being offered for "general maintenance". Another supplement says on the box cover that it is "twice as strong to reduce menopausal symptoms" and its use is listed as to "help reduce hot flashes and night sweats" – nothing in the way of support or maintenance. Structure and functions claims are not approved or preapproved by FDA. However, the marketer must notify FDA of the structure and function claims it will be making within 30 days of marketing. And the marketer, not FDA, is responsible for the validity of the claims. When a supplement includes a structure and function claim on its label, the label must by law also include the statement, "This statement has not been evaluated by the Food and Drug Administration. This product is not intended to diagnose, treat or prevent any disease." The second sentence is required because only a drug can make such claims and this statement is intended to say that these supplements/nutriceuticals are not drugs. This fine point may be missed by most of the public, and there seems to be no shortage of patient self- treatment with supplements. The issue of why people are taking supplements, especially those making structure and function claims, when supplements cannot treat or prevent any disease is officially answered with the notion that the supplements help the body maintain its healthy steady state. To comply with this aim and avoid drug claims, most of the structure and function claims are oriented around the idea that the supplement is allowing the tissue to maintain its healthy state. However, when read critically most of these statements are nonsensical, especially to the medical mind.

In addition to structure and function claims, there are two other categories of claims which can be made for dietary supplements: health claims and nutrient content claims. Health claims describe the relationship between dietary supplements and reducing the risk of disease. One of the following three conditions is needed in order to make a health claim about a supplement:

1. FDA must have already authorized the claim;
2. A U.S. government or a National Academy of Science scientific body must have issued a statement on the relationship; or
3. There must be enough emerging evidence to allow a restricted health claim, called a "qualified health claim."

The third type of allowable claim, nutrient content claims, are very limited and may only be made based on FDA authorizing regulations. Nutrient content claims allow the label to state the level of a nutrient or dietary substance and use terms such as "free", "high", "low", "more", "reduced" and "lite".

As regards the safety of supplements, the company which manufactures or distributes the supplements is responsible for the agent's safety and must have evidence to support that their claims are not misleading or false. Unless the supplements contain ingredients not in the food chain before 1994, companies do not need FDA approval to sell/market a supplement. Supplements containing *new dietary ingredients,* i.e., since 1994, cannot be marketed without FDA approval of safety and other information. However, since passage of the DSHEA in 1994 over 50,000 new supplements have been marketed. Although it is not known how many of these new supplements contain novel or post-1994 new dietary ingredients, FDA has received less than 200 adequate notifications for the safety of new dietary ingredients.

Overall, supplements as we know them are allowed on the market because of laws passed by Congress in response to popular pressure in favor of the dietary supplements. The supplements clearly tend to run counter to FDA's policies requiring high levels of scientific documentation as to safety and efficacy. Although FDA approval is not required before marketing, except for supplements containing new dietary ingredients, FDA can inspect the manufacturing sites and follow up on complaints. In a 3-year study ending in 2012, FDA inspectors cited 70 % of over 600 manufacturers for manufacturing issues such as failure to keep proper sanitation and failure to document ingredients. Separately there have been numerous instances of supplements being adulterated, i.e., containing unlabeled and/or unsafe ingredients. For example, in the past few years according to FDA, manufacturers have voluntarily recalled more than 80 bodybuilding supplements because they were found to contain synthetic steroids or steroid-like substances, 50 sexual-enhancement products that contained sildenafil (Viagra) or other erectile-dysfunction drugs and 40 weight-loss supplements containing sibutramine (Meridia) and other drugs. There are currently numerous calls for repeal of the Dietary Supplement Act, which many, including most physicians, probably consider to have been a failed experiment.

Chapter 7
What Are Cosmetics and Cosmeceuticals?

FDA defines cosmetics as articles applied topically for beautifying, promoting attractiveness, altering the appearance or cleansing. For FDA the difference between a cosmetic and a drug is its intended use. The intended use of a drug is to diagnose, cure, mitigate, treat or prevent a disease, or to affect the structure or function of the body. When an article claims to restore hair growth or take away varicose veins it is making drug, not cosmetic, claims. Using agents such as fluoride in toothpaste, which is known to have therapeutic effects, also indicates a drug rather than a cosmetic intent. For example, toothpastes containing fluorides are regulated as non-prescription, that is OTC Anticaries Drug Products. Even the perception by the buying public that a product has a therapeutic effect may indicate intent consistent with a drug. When the intended use is solely for beautifying, cleansing, promoting attractiveness and so forth, an agent is a cosmetic and as such is not subject to pre-marketing approval by FDA. The cosmetic firms have the ultimate responsibility for substantiation of a cosmetic product's safety.

Many products have both a cosmetic and drug intent. For example, a shampoo is a cosmetic because it is intended to clean hair. However, an antidandruff shampoo is also a drug because its intended use is the treatment of a disease. Other examples of articles which are both a cosmetic and a drug are moisturizers and make-up with sun protection claims, and deodorants that are also antiperspirants. When a product is a combination of a cosmetic and drug it must comply with both the drug and the cosmetic regulations and would therefore require pre-market approval as a drug. (In most cases the drug approval is by way of the monograph.) In addition to not being able to make drug claims, for cosmetics there are no provisions for structure and function claims, health claims or nutrient claims, all of which are available for nutritional supplements.

Although pre-market approval is not required to sell cosmetics, it is not fair to say that cosmetic products are unregulated. Cosmetics are regulated by FDA's Center for Food Safety and Applied Nutrition which is responsible for cosmetic products being safe and properly labeled. FDA requires that cosmetics be unadulterated, not misbranded and contain an ingredients label. Physicians may not realize

© Springer International Publishing Switzerland 2014
W.H. Eaglstein, *The FDA for Doctors*, DOI 10.1007/978-3-319-08362-9_7

that these terms, "adulterated" and "misbranded", are very broad in reach. For example, in addition to adulteration referring to the cosmetic containing filthy, putrid, or decomposed substances, it also means containing any poisonous substance or material that, when the product is used as intended, is dangerous. Adulteration applies not only to the product itself but also to the container and the environment in which the cosmetic is manufactured. Misbranded refers not only to false and misleading labeling, but the absence of a label, the failure to offer the required information or even to a damaged label. Labeling refers to all written, printed, or graphic matter on or accompanying a product, and misbranding is also considered to occur when labels are difficult to read. Even misleading packaging can be considered misbranding.

Doctors might well agree that these regulatory requirements are insufficient from some points of view and FDA seems to agree, in that FDA does not allow cosmetics to be labeled "FDA Approved" even when the cosmetic has complied not only with the requirements mentioned above but also with certain voluntary registration requirements developed by FDA. In addition to there being no pre-market approval requirement for cosmetics, there is no requirement to substantiate product safety, no requirement to keep or report serious adverse effects or to register facilities. FDA does not have recall authority for cosmetics but does ask companies to voluntarily recall products and assists with such recalls.

Because of the perceived shortcomings of FDA authority and regulation of cosmetics, many states, most conspicuously California, have developed their own additional regulations on cosmetics sold in their state. These regulations have largely been in response to concerned non-governmental organizations having raised many issues, such as phthalates in cosmetics reducing serum testosterone levels and causing birth defects; formaldehyde releasers in cosmetics causing cancers; and cosmetic face paints containing the toxin lead. The proliferation of different state regulations have led to proposals by the cosmetic industry that FDA's regulatory authority be strengthened and that FDA's regulations supplant or override any state authority.

Finally, cosmeceuticals, which are topically-applied combinations of cosmetics and ingredients thought to have biologic activity for which there is theoretic or in vitro evidence that a drug-like effect might be produced, are not a regulatory category recognized by FDA. Because the name "cosmeceuticals", a combination of cosmetics and pharmaceutics, suggests that the agents have drug- like activity, critics complain that users are misled into believing the agents are active and somehow approved by FDA. Certainly much of the packaging and promotional pieces fortify that impression. For example, on the website of one such product, listed below the title "The Science Behind....." the following are listed: "clinical trials showed lipopeptide firmed the skin by up to 40 %"; "natural protein isolate was shown to help the skin appear more firm and lifted"; "tripeptide helps skin appear denser, firmer and smoother"; "a significant smoothing and anti-wrinkle effect was seen after 84 days of twice daily application"; "ceramide/peptide pairing has been shown to reduce the appearance of fine lines and wrinkles"; "biotechnological extract smoothness, roughness and crepiness"; "clinical studies showed a decrease in the appearance of wrinkle depth." Another product states that "a proprietary blend of Bamboo, Silica, English Pea Extract and Glucosamine has been shown to hydrate, firm and tone skin, and antioxidants, Vitamins C and E, help skin appear brighter and more even-toned." That many such agents are sold in doctors' offices, sometimes exclusively so, further fortifies the idea to patients that they are products containing active agents.

The agents added to the cosmeceuticals, fall into categories such as antioxidants, claimed to reduce aging; retinol, claimed to have anti-wrinkle activities as found with retinoic acid; peptides, alleged to stimulate skin collagen production; and growth factors, which can stimulate cell division and vessel proliferation in vitro. These cosmeceutical products are often very expensive and beautifully packaged. However, just as FDA does not recognize the category of oral agents known as nutriceuticals, or nutritional supplements which might produce drug-like effects, FDA does not recognize the category of cosmeceuticals. Interestingly, in some countries cosmetics with mildly active additives are a recognized category.

Chapter 8
What Is the FDA and What Does It Do?

The FDA is a part of the Executive or Presidential branch of the U.S. Federal Government. It is one of 11 operating agencies in the Department of Health and Human Services (HHS). Among the HHS operating agencies best known to physicians, are the NIH (National Institute of Health), the CDC (Centers for Disease Control and Prevention) and CMS (Centers for Medicare and Medicaid Service Services). In broad terms FDA's mission is to protect and promote the public health by regulating and supervising the nation's food supply, tobacco products, dietary supplements, human and veterinary drugs, vaccines, biopharmaceuticals, blood transfusions and medical devices including electromagnetic radiation emitting devices. Of interest is that FDA does not regulate meat and poultry both of which are regulated by the Department of Agriculture (FDA was once part of the Department of Agriculture), water, except bottled water, and alcohol. As noted earlier, for doctors it is important to realize that FDA regulates medical products – not medical practices or the practice of medicine which is regulated by the states. Also as noted elsewhere, although FDA regulates the sale of instruments used in surgery, the surgical procedures themselves are not regulated by FDA.

Since FDA is part of the Executive Branch, the President appoints the head of the FDA, the FDA Commissioner, with the advice and consent of the Congress. Organizationally it is composed of a number of Centers and Offices (Table 8.1). The Centers of most concern to doctors are those which regulate drugs, biologicals and devices: the Center for Drug Evaluation and Research (CDER), the Center for Biologics Evaluation and Research (CBER) and the Center for Devices and Radiological Health (CDRH). FDA headquarters are in a suburb of Washington D.C., White Oak, Maryland, and most of its meetings which are of interest to doctors are held in and around Washington, D.C. There are also over 150 field offices and a number of laboratories which are dispersed around the U.S., the Virgin Islands and Puerto Rico. FDA also has offices in foreign countries, where more and more manufacturing facilities require inspections. Overall about one-third of the agency's employees are stationed outside of the Washington, D.C. area, staffing five regional

© Springer International Publishing Switzerland 2014
W.H. Eaglstein, *The FDA for Doctors*, DOI 10.1007/978-3-319-08362-9_8

Table 8.1 FDA is an agency within the Department of Health and Human Services[1] and consists of nine Centers and Offices

Executive branch of the government
Department of Health and Human Services (also NIH, CDC, CMS and HIS)
Food and Drug Administration
Center for Drug Evaluation and Research
Center for Biologics Evaluation and Research
Center for Devices and Radiologic Health
Center for veterinary Medicine
National Center for Toxicological Research

Those of most import to doctors are listed above
NIH National Institutes of Health, *CDC* Centers for Disease Control and Prevention, *CMS* Center for Medicare and Medicaid Services, *HIS* Indian Health Services

Table 8.2 FDA budget and employees

Fiscal year	$ millions
2006	1,972
2012	3,800
2013	4,500

Approx. 15,000 Employees (2013)

offices, 20 district offices, field offices and laboratories. FDA inspectors and scientists visit and inspect some 16,000 facilities a year and also cooperate with similar state activities.

FDA's regulatory jurisdiction is so broad that it is estimated to encompass 25 cents of every dollar Americans spend. FDA has only about 15,000 employees and a budget of about $4.5 billion (Table 8.2). Clearly, this budget and number of employees is too small to actively police a consequential portion of the activities associated with 25 % of all American expenditures, so the system necessarily depends a great deal on voluntary self-regulation. From time to time FDA prosecutes or takes enforcement actions with the broad aim of obtaining a great deal of publicity about an issue which it is hoped will serve to fortify the appropriate self-regulation.

Until the 1992 imposition of "User Fees" (a fee charged for the use of a public service or product), the entire budget for drug regulation was derived from Congress. User Fees, which were originally only charged to those applying for drug approval, are now also charged for biologics and devices. They are fees which the sponsors pay to have their drug or device regulated (evaluated and approved or disapproved for marketing). For many years the imposition by FDA of User Fees were resisted on the grounds that the fees would make the agency dependent upon the entities they regulated. Since those regulated would be providing the funds for the required regulation, it would be a classic case of the fox guarding the chicken coop. Nevertheless, by 1992 the time between a drug's approval in foreign markets and its approval in the U.S., known as the "drug lag", was perceived to be so great that Congress approved the imposition of user fees with passage of the Prescription

Drug User Fee Act (PDUFA), which has been subsequently broadened and renewed several times. User Fees now account for nearly one-half of FDA's budget, the other half coming from the Federal Budget.

For an idea of what is charged for User Fees, in FY 2010 a new drug application user fee was between $500,000 and $3.2 million depending upon the level of data submitted, while a biologic license could cost up to $5.9 million. Reduced fee arrangements are provided for new and small companies. These fees are for review and do not assure approval. The User Fee revenues, which have allowed FDA to hire more reviewers and improve systems, have been remarkably successful at speeding product approval. In contrast to the drug lag occurring before the User Fee imposition, the U.S. review time and approval time is now faster than that in many other advanced nations. Doctors and the public are frequently told of the many years needed to develop a drug, on average 12 for a new chemical entity. While the user fee revenues have reduced the review time from about 2 years to 1 year, reviews of applications will usually only start after the completion of the years of work necessary to develop the information needed for application and approval. Such work is unaffected by the faster review time. However, a 1-year reduction in the review time can result in earlier approval and marketing, which, considering the revenues afforded by many new drugs, is very valuable and is the reason that drug developers willingly supported and in fact lobbied to have the imposition of User Fees.

As noted in earlier sections, the FDA and its activities is a vast subject engaging thousands of lawyers, regulators, scientists, physicians, writers, legislators and many others directly and indirectly. And although much of the core information upon which FDA makes decisions is based on scientific knowledge and medical practice activities, in fact, FDA's existence and powers rest on legislative constructs and laws which reflect broad societal judgments and political pressures, which are often far removed from the everyday practice of medicine.

Chapter 9
Foods, Doctors and the FDA

FDA is responsible for assuring the safety, security and accurate labeling of the nation's food supply. As noted elsewhere, FDA regulates goods that constitute about 25 % of all U.S. expenditures, and foods account for about three-quarters of the total value of goods regulated by FDA. As such, FDA enforces regulations which apply from "farm to fork", including over $400 billion worth of domestic food, about $50 billion worth of imported foods, and over $60 billion worth of cosmetics sold across state lines. The FDA Center for Food Safety and Applied Nutrition is responsible for carrying out FDA's food mission which is to promote and protect the public's health by ensuring that the nation's food supply is safe, sanitary, wholesome, and honestly labeled. Surprisingly, the Center is also responsible for ensuring that cosmetic products are safe and properly labeled. For FDA the term "food" means (1) articles used for food or drink for man or other animals; (2) chewing gum; and (3) articles used for components of any such article. FDA is also in charge of all food additives, for example, preservatives added to extend the shelf life of prepared foods. There are, however, some important and not obvious exceptions to FDA's food jurisdiction. For example, most meats and meat-containing products are regulated by the Department of Agriculture, which also shares regulatory authority over eggs. However, exotic meats (game) and seafood are under FDA as are dietary supplements. Other federal agencies also have some responsibility for regulation of food products. For example, the United State Environment Protection Agency (EPA) regulates levels of allowable contaminants in public drinking water, whereas FDA regulates bottled water.

Overall, through the Center, FDA's food safety concerns are very broad in nature and include issues such as naturally occurring toxins , e.g. ciguatera toxin, pesticide residues, toxic metals such as lead or mercury, and radionuclides in addition to the more common problems of bacterial contamination and filth, e.g., insect and rodent fragments and droppings, and product tampering. Among the methods FDA has for protecting the food supply are inspection, including collection and analysis of samples from establishments; monitoring of food and cosmetic imports; monitoring of adverse event reports and consumer complaints; developing and improving methods

© Springer International Publishing Switzerland 2014
W.H. Eaglstein, *The FDA for Doctors*, DOI 10.1007/978-3-319-08362-9_9

for determining pathogen and chemical contamination of foods (and cosmetics); and studying the effects of processing on foods.

Importantly, FDA publishes a list of ingredients which are "generally regarded as safe" – so called, GRAS chemicals, which may be added to foods and containers for foods without pre-market approval. There are about 500 such chemicals on the FDA GRAS list. As might be expected, regulations encompassing a large part of the food chain are complex. What might seem simple, such as knowing which chemicals are considered safe for our foods, is not easily known and frequently has not been formally studied. For example, some chemicals are allowed based the their having been safely a part of the food chain for extended periods while others are allowed because they are on the GRAS list. When manufacturers want to have a chemical additive considered to be GRAS, they must develop the scientific basis for such a designation, including formation of panels of experts to assert the status to FDA. Importantly, the GRAS designation is to be for the additive's intended use rather than for all usages. FDA may have the request under review for long periods of time and ultimately, rather than confirming the GRAS designation, FDA issues a "no comment" letter implying that no challenge will be made and thus confirming the GRAS status. Alternatively, FDA may reject the claim. Even the types of materials upon which foods are processed are regulated by FDA. Finally, food labeling such as the ingredients list and the nutrition facts are regulated as part of FDA's food safety goal. From time to time FDA updates the labeling format for food, especially those that are processed, as part of its effort to give the public sufficient information to avoid obesity and other current public health concerns.

Dietary supplements and so called nutriceuticals (see Chap. 6) are products that contain concentrated ingredients derived from food. By law, a dietary ingredient must be one or a combination of compounds such as vitamins, minerals, herbs or other botanicals and amino acids. FDA regulates dietary supplements in accordance with a special law known as the Dietary Supplement Health and Education Act passed in 1994. This act was created because of popular pressure, and in the name of deregulation restricted FDA from exerting drug authority over supplements as long as manufacturers made no claims about preventing or treating disease. As a result, FDA currently regulates dietary supplements as a category of food, and not as drugs. For supplements containing dietary ingredients in the food chain before 1994 companies are not required to have premarketing approval from FDA. According to the Act, companies selling supplements are responsible for determining that their products are safe and for determining that there is adequate evidence to substantiate structure and function claims about the supplements. To deal with safety issues, the 1994 legislation requires the FDA to demonstrate that individual supplements are unsafe using its adverse events reporting system, which may capture only 1–10 % of all adverse events linked to supplements. Since dietary supplements are not drugs and not approved by FDA, all supplements carry a boxed statement to the effect that the supplements are not approved by FDA and are not for the diagnosis, treatment or preventions of diseases or conditions. (See Chap. 6 for a more complete discussion of Supplements and Nutraceuticals).

Chapter 10
The FDA Approval Process and Drug Development

Overview

Drug development is governed by a so-called "iron triangle" made up of the need for intellectual property (patents), financial return on investment and regulatory approval. As mentioned earlier, by FDA approval we really mean approval to market, or enter into interstate commerce, often called pre-market approval since the approval must be obtained before a drug can be marketed. Importantly, FDA does not regulate the practice of medicine. Many physicians as well as a considerable portion of the public believe that FDA regulates what doctors can do. Upon reflection physicians realize that their license to practice medicine is issued by states and that generally it is the state that regulates the practice of medicine. Obviously, if an agent is not available for a physician to use because it is not approved for marketing by the FDA then our ability to practice, at least with that agent, is curtailed.

For most types of drugs – prescription drugs, biologics and other FDA drug regulatory categories such as botanical drugs, non-prescription drugs and so forth – there are well developed pre-market approval requirements. Perhaps the best developed of these approval pathways and the one usually considered most demanding is the New Drug Application (NDA) pathway. This pathway will be the template and the core of the discussion in this chapter. The pre-market requirements and processes for devices have become much better defined over the past two decades but are less demanding than those for drugs. The approval process for cosmetics and supplements requires far less effort in the active sense, with the ultimate regulatory requirement emphasizing what cannot be claimed. Also, activities such as surgery itself are not regulated by FDA. That is, the surgical procedure is not subject to FDA regulation although the devices, from scalpels and other instruments which are used to do surgery, are regulated, as are the many devices which are implanted.

The initial FDA pre-market approval process (1938) focused on and required only that drugs be safe. It was generally felt that physicians and patients would be able to determine the utility or efficacy of drugs. Although Thalidomide was never approved by the FDA and was never sold in the United States, the birth defects that

© Springer International Publishing Switzerland 2014
W.H. Eaglstein, *The FDA for Doctors*, DOI 10.1007/978-3-319-08362-9_10

thalidomide caused in Europe alarmed the U.S. population so much that congress passed a comprehensive FDA reform bill readdressing the need for safety. This legislation, passed in 1962 and known as the Kefauver-Harris Drug Amendments, added the requirement that drugs be proved effective in addition to safe before they could be marketed. Since then (1962), all drugs have been required to be proved both safe and effective before approval for marketing (pre-market approval). Most of the drugs and other agents that were already on the market before the 1962 requirement to prove efficacy were reviewed by FDA-appointed panels and were approved based on available efficacy data or asked to generate new data or be removed from the market. A few agents were never reviewed and form the basis of the so-called DESI (Drug Efficacy Safety Investigation) drug category. It was only in 1976 that the medical device amendments requiring pre-market approval of devices, including diagnostic products, was enacted by Congress.

To satisfy the safety and efficacy pre-market requirements, sponsors (usually pharmaceutical companies) test drugs by a variety of methods, including chemical and physical assays, bioassays, cell, tissue and animal model evaluations, and finally, human trials. For a New Drug Application (NDA), involving a new chemical entity (NCE) the process is quite costly, up to an estimated $800 million, and takes about 15 years, which is double the time needed in 1964. The aim of an NDA is to give FDA enough information for FDA to determine if the proposed new drug is safe and effective for its proposed use(s), and to decide whether the benefits of using the drug the outweigh the risks. Not readily appreciated by physicians is the intensity with which the proposed drug label is also evaluated for approval. The final label is usually the result of a significant negotiation between FDA and the sponsor, and includes all information allowed by FDA. Even less often considered by the medical community is that the sponsor must submit evidence that the proposed drug can be manufactured properly, with controls to assure consistent drug quality, and that the proposed drug must be able to preserve its identity, strength and purity under conditions of storage and distribution before it is used.

In reality, the cost of generating sufficient information for an NDA or other approval varies a great deal. The wide range in development costs reflects not only the variations inherent in the type of drug and the sponsor's efficiency, but also a variety of accounting methodologies. For example, the cost of developing a drug with a novel new chemical entity as the active agent will be greater than the cost of developing a new formulation using an already marketed active pharmaceutical ingredient. The cost of developing topically applied drugs is less than that for systemically administered drugs. And of course the cost of developing a generic drug is below the cost of developing an original or reference listed drug. As regards accounting for the cost of development, the cost of being able to develop drugs includes the costs of developing drugs that make it to market, the winners, and the cost of losers, or drugs that fail at some point in the development process – the vast majority. Therefore, the costs of the losers are typically added as a cost of developing the "winners." Other factors accounting for the wide range of development costs include whether the cited cost is in pre-tax or after tax dollars, and whether there is inclusion of lost interest income on the dollars invested in the development process.

It is of course fair to say that NCEs can cost hundreds of millions to develop but other categories of drugs, for example topicals using known systemic active pharmaceutical agents (APIs), may cost in the range of $30–50 million.

Because drug development is such a costly process it will rarely be undertaken unless some form of patent protection exists for the ultimate drug product. Patents are also known as intellectual property because they are a government granted and protected method of owning ideas. Patents come in several forms. The most desirable protection is a patent on the API or drug substance, known as a Composition of Matter Patent. However, other levels of patent protection also exist, such as a patent on the method of manufacture, a Methods Patent, or a patent on the specific use, such as the drug's use in a certain disease, a so-called Use Patent. In the U.S., initial patent protection is for 20 years. Since in almost all cases serious amounts of money will not be spent on development unless there is patent protection, the patent will be issued before development proceeds very far. Because the development process, in particular complying with the clinical studies portion of the FDA pre-market approval process, will then consume a significant number of the years of protection afforded by the patent, there is in place a method to "extend" or give back some of these years of patent exclusivity, dependent partially upon the number of years required to get FDA approval. This is the so-called Patent Restoration Act. The total amount of time restored cannot exceed 5 years. As noted elsewhere, devices cost far less to develop. This is especially true for Class I devices and Class II devices using the 510K route.

Although implied, it is important to recognize that the studies and other investigations involved with the development of a drug or other agent are carried out by the sponsor. FDA may offer guidance on studies or other works the agency believes will be needed for approval, but the work is done by the sponsor, most often a drug or device company.

Finally, as regards return on investment, it is important to realize how difficult it is to development a new chemical entity. Although statistics vary depending upon the analysis, in general, for every 10,000 chemicals screened, 250 are studied pre-clinically, 5 reach Phase 2 clinical trials and one reaches the market (Fig. 10.1). For at least two decades, major drug development companies have been heavily dependent on so-called blockbuster drugs, that is, drugs with sales of over $1 billion per year. Many blockbusters produce sales of $3 billion or more per year and represent well over 10 % of a company's annual revenues. The revenues of these drugs are very important to companies and of course are alleged to be the reason companies can continue to put large sums into developing new agents. Companies are criticized for spending more on advertisements than research but it is hard to get doctors to change prescribing habits even in order to offer their patients advanced drug therapy. To continue to receive these revenues companies resort to a number of strategies such as patenting variations of the blockbuster drug – the companies are criticized for the creation of these me-too drugs – which the company hopes will continue to produce the high revenues after the patent on the original drug expires. When many blockbuster drugs are to go off patent at about the same time, it is often referred to as a patent cliff. When drugs go off patent, generic manufacturers produce generic

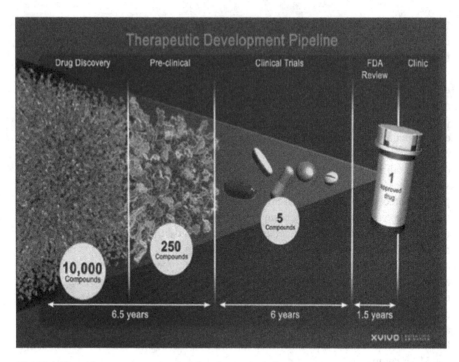

Fig. 10.1 One of many schematics showing the number of attempts for each successful new drug

versions of the original, or pioneer, drug. Although the first generic manufacturer does make considerable money on their product, ultimately within about 2 years the generic versions of the original blockbuster are selling for approximately 20 % of the initial price when the drug was patent protected. Obviously, one can see how it is that without patent protection companies might not undertake the costly process of drug development. In the past 15 years, drugs for rare diseases, or orphan drugs, have been the focus of considerable interest by drug development companies. This is because the development of these agents is given some preferential treatment by FDA, and once developed the market is usually found to be much larger than the less than 200,000 affected people or potential patients required for orphan drug status. Importantly, because these drugs are usually singular for the rare disease, insurance companies will pay especially high prices for them. Drugs to treat lethal cancers are another area in which the return on investment has been especially attractive because of the high likelihood that insurers and individuals will pay high prices for these life-extending if not life-saving drugs. However, in general drug developers must cope with the issue of whether a drug they are considering developing will have a market or financial return which is large enough to justify the development costs, which also include returns sufficient to pay for losers and other ongoing expenses. This calculation is obviously complex and even more so if the drug is truly unique because in that case the size of the market is especially conjectural.

Preclinical Testing

Preclinical testing might refer to any study done before studies in humans (clinical testing), but is usually considered to be those studies done after identification of a potential drug, or drug candidate. Often the idea for a potential drug intervention, especially a novel intervention, emanates from basic science observations or study results generated by laboratory scientists. The basic science laboratory observations are utilized as an assay system to empirically evaluate thousands of chemicals to see if they affect the assay in such a way as to possibly be useful as a drug. This approach is called high throughput screening and the thousands of chemicals evaluated are known as libraries. However, regardless of the process whereby a candidate drug is identified, the process of taking candidate drugs from the basic science laboratory to the bedside requires work which is very different from the type of exploratory basic studies which often initiated the candidate discovery process.

Among the first requirements for developing a drug are a number of processes or steps which collectively are referred to as CMC which stands for Chemistry, Manufacturing and Control. In these processes the physicochemical properties of the potential drug are determined. In addition to knowing or determining precisely the drug candidate's chemical makeup/structure, its solubility and other physical properties, especially its stability over time, are determined. The methods for manufacturing the drug candidate need to be refined to insure a consistent product, and as the drug development proceeds the ability to make a small amount for initial testing needs to expand so that ultimately amounts large enough for human testing and then for marketing can be made.

The process of moving from the reproducible production of small amounts to a large amount is known as "scaling-up" and generally problems arise at each increase in scale, all of which need to be overcome to ensure in each instance that the same product is produced. Of course in the early CMC phase it is necessary to develop the active agent appropriately for use in pills, capsules, aerosol, IV, topical and other routes of administration. Its purity (including microbiologic purity), stability, consistency and durability (shelf–life) need to be determined. Problems are encountered at all stages of these early processes and many times account for failure to go forward with development. These are issues which are key to drug developers and regulators but which are rarely considered by physicians. As noted earlier, these are important steps in the development process but are not at all similar to the basic science work which often underlies the entire effort. Neither the work nor the people carrying out the work are the same.

In concert with the early CMC activities are in vitro and animal studies of a compound's pharmacology and toxicity. These studies include animal studies of its bioactivity (pharmacodynamics), metabolism (pharmacokinetics) and mechanism-of-action, and hence its potential usefulness. In vitro and in vivo systems help define both its potential efficacies and toxicities. It is not usually realized by physicians that many of the preclinical toxicity studies are performed at higher and higher doses in order to deliberately reach toxicity and thereby understand the toxicities agents can produce, e.g., affecting the heart or impacting the liver, which should ultimately be looked for in human testing and use. In fact, an agent for which some toxicity cannot be induced should be suspected of being biologically inactive rather than extremely safe.

Although there are now tests for toxicity that can be done using in vitro methods, e.g., with isolated cells and organ cultures, most tests for toxicity must still be done with experimental animals, which allow confidence that the interaction of a full immune and metabolic system with the test agent can be assessed. For all drug candidates animal testing will usually be done in two small animal species using short term exposures and escalating doses. In certain circumstances tests might even need to be done in primates. For agents anticipated to be used chronically or for short time periods but repetitively, chronic dosing studies are usually required. If there is the possibility that the potential drug might cause cancer, special studies in animals designed to detect cancer producing activities may be required. Although, in general, preclinical testing is considered to be inexpensive, especially relative to the cost of human clinical trials such as those done in Phases 2 and 3, chronic treatment studies in animals, such as those done to evaluate an agent for topical photocarcinogenesis, can be quite costly, easily reaching the range of $1 million and may take from several months to 2 years to carry out.

Clinical Testing

Clinical (human) testing is conducted in sequential dependent phases called Phases 1, 2, 3, and 4. However, there is also a little used, so-called Phase 0 stage of human testing in which greatly reduced, sub-therapeutic single doses of the potential drug are administered to a very few volunteers, 5–15, with the aim of studying the compound's pharmacodynamics (how the drug works in the body) and/or pharmacokinetics (how the body processes the drug). Phase 0 studies are also known as human micro dosing studies. While Phase 0 studies are first-in-human studies, they are not designed to gain information on efficacy or safety. Although they might be valuable in the development process, they are infrequently used or written about.

Legally the FDA requirement for efficacy calls for "substantial" evidence of efficacy shown through controlled clinical trials. Safety is considered to be demonstration in controlled trials that the drug benefits outweigh the risks and that the drug may be labeled in a fashion suitable for safe use. The safety consideration obviously leaves room for the use of drugs that are not actually safe but are considered worth it relative to the potential benefit and the risk of no treatment. Obtaining the information needed to allow FDA to make these determinations comes in considerable measure from the Phase 1, 2 and 3 studies.

Phase 1 studies deal with safety, Phase 2 with safety and efficacy at different doses, Phase 3 with safety and efficacy using the drug dosage to be marketed and in sufficient numbers of patients to allow a determination regarding final marketing approval, while Phase 4 studies are post-marketing studies done with an already approved drug.

For every 5,000–10,000 pharmaceutical compounds evaluated or screened, about five reach the stage of clinical trials and only about one of these five actually reaches the market after FDA approval (Fig. 10.1). Of those compounds failing in clinical trials, about 37 % fail in Phase 1, 50 % fail in Phase 2, and 13 % fail in Phase 3. The sponsors conduct and pay for those studies needed to prove safety and efficacy. The FDA evaluates and judges the test results, but rarely does drug testing. However, the FDA is involved in the sponsor's test plans, especially in the plans allowing human testing. Technically, the FDA controls only the right to market a drug or regulated medical device via interstate commerce. That is, the FDA controls the right to pass a drug through interstate commerce, but does not regulate the practice of medicine. At least in theory a drug not approved by FDA could be manufactured and sold within a state and could be tested in humans and or used medically within a state. Such tests would, however, most likely be subject to state and institutional approval, which would be difficult to obtain without an FDA exemption.

Because potential new drugs (investigational drugs) have not been proved safe and effective, they may not be given as therapy and the sponsor, usually through clinical investigators not employed full time by the sponsor, may give the investigational drug to people for evaluation (testing) only after obtaining FDA approval by way of an application known as an Investigative New Drug exemption, or IND. The IND is an exemption allowing interstate shipment of and human administration of a "drug" not known to be safe or effective in order that it may be tested in humans. When a company or an investigator wants to begin clinical testing they submit the IND which has the results of animal testing, drug production and the test protocol for FDA approval. The company may proceed with the protocol testing 30 days after submission to FDA. That is, FDA has 30 days in which to ask that the testing not proceed, usually asking for more information and time for further evaluation of the application. The IND mechanism is also such that FDA does not actively approve but rather fails to stop the testing.

The aim of clinical trials or drug trials is to study the drug rather than to treat a patient. That is to say, even patients in a clinical trial are really volunteers for testing a drug, and in fact a drug trial need not be done by a physician since the investigator is not practicing medicine but rather studying a drug. In practice, usually the investigators for most drug trials are licensed physicians. However, it is important to appreciate that physicians conducting a drug trial or study are generally "required" to act within or follow a written protocol, rather than adjusting therapy to the individual patient's or participant's circumstances. Because of these restrictions many physicians are not able to be, or not comfortable being study doctors.

The results of studies done under an IND are ultimately a part of the NDA for obtaining approval. There are exceptions to the requirement that agents not be used for treatment unless they have been proved to be safe and effective. Chief among these exceptions is the regulation allowing a so called "treatment IND" which allows an experimental drug which shows promise in clinical testing, to be used to treat serious or immediately life-threatening conditions before the final clinical work on the drug is conducted and the FDA review takes place. Another exception is the allowance of a so-called Emergency Use IND under which the FDA authorizes use of an experimental drug in an emergency situation that does not allow time for submission of an IND.

Phase 1 Testing

In Phase 1, healthy volunteers or patients receive the drug in order to study its safety, along with its metabolic (pharmacokinetic) and pharmacologic (pharmacodynamic) profiles. For tests of a new molecular entity, Phase 1 trials are frequently called "first in human" trials. Usually, Phase 1 testing involves 20–80 volunteers, and the safety testing is general as well as specific, depending upon the toxicities detected in animal studies. The Phase 1 drug safety study volunteers are most often healthy young people, despite the fact that a high percentage of medicines are ultimately taken by older and often quite ill patients. Drugs aimed at late stage cancer or certain lethal infectious diseases such as advanced HIV are likely to be tested on patients rather than healthy volunteers, especially when the drug is likely to make the subjects ill. Most Phase 1 testing is done by commercial organizations specializing in such work and known as contract research organizations (CROs). The volunteers are normally observed for several drug half-lives and depending on the nature of the drug they may stay at the facility throughout all or much of the testing.

Phase 1 is intended to give enough safety, pharmacokinetic and pharmacologic information to allow the design of controlled clinical studies to be done in Phase 2. Often Phase 1 studies are designed so that one or two subjects take a very low dose, e.g., one-tenth the dose which produced no observable adverse effects in an appropriate animal. Once ascertained to be safe at such vary low dosage, an additional group is dosed at a higher level and so forth. The same ascending dose approach can be used with multiple rather than single doses. Usually a placebo control group is included to give a baseline to allow the evaluation of side effects found in the testing circumstances. Blood, urine and other testing, including in certain circumstances tissue sampling, for example to try to detect the drug's action on cancer cells, will be done through the course of the Phase 1 trial. Importantly, Phase 1 should generate an early but clear idea of acute side effects and other toxicities. For oral agents, studies of the effects of food on absorption will also be done this phase. As mentioned, Phase 1 study results allow the protocol to be developed for Phase 2 trials.

Phase 2 Testing

In Phase 2 clinical studies, the drug is tested for safety and efficacy in a still fairly limited number (usually several hundred) of volunteers who have the condition the drug is aimed at treating. Phase 2 is often thought of as having two substages, Phases

2a and 2b. Phase 2a studies will be smaller or pilot studies aimed at confirming the drug concept and predicting dosage. Often sponsors want to meet with FDA after successful 2a studies to confirm that their plans for the larger and more costly 2b studies seem suitable to FDA. Phase 2b studies are expected to explore different doses for both efficacy and safety. Three doses are commonly studied. The aim is to identify a dose close to the lowest dose that is optimally effective so as to not give people more of a drug than is needed. These studies will ordinarily be double-blinded with the control being either a placebo or comparator standard-of-care treatment drug. As mentioned elsewhere, it is important to understand that the FDA requirement that a drug be effective and safe is interpreted to mean compared to a placebo treatment. In Europe and elsewhere, new drugs must prove to be equal to or better than the standard treatment.

Phase 2 studies are expected to define the conditions which will then be tested in larger studies aimed at "proving" safety and efficacy for defined conditions (diseases) in defined populations. As an aside, we physicians often use drugs for indications in which the drug was not studied, i.e., a different population or indication. We make the assumption that the now approved drug we use in a new population will be safe since it was safe in the approval studies for the currently indicated population. This sort of off-label use is important for us and our patients, seems reasonable and usually is without obvious problem. However, FDA does not assume usage in a new population/new indication will be safe (or effective) and requires additional studies before approving such.

Because Phase 2 studies are done to select the most appropriate dose and conditions for final or Phase 3 testing, the efficacy endpoints used in Phase 2 studies are sometimes less definitive, e.g., a surrogate endpoint, than the end point ultimately required by FDA for Phase 3 studies and approval. Phase 2 is the point in the clinical development pathway that most drug development failure occurs. The Phase 2 failure rate is 50–70 % depending upon the analysis. The failure is as likely to be due to safety concerns as it is to inadequate efficacy. Although uncommon, very successful Phase 2 results, for drugs aimed at treating serious or life-threatening diseases may be sufficient for FDA approval. Usually approvals of drugs based on work ending with Phase 2 study results, will also require that Phase 3 type trials ultimately, be done and be successful. FDA's withdrawal of bevacizumab (Avastin) for breast cancer after Phase 3 type tests done after marketing did not reproduce the benefit that the drug had shown in Phase 2 studies is an example of this requirement and the consequences of failure in such studies done after marketing.

Phase 3 Testing

Phase 3 studies are aimed at providing sufficient safety and efficacy information to allow FDA to approve the drug for marketing. Phase 3 studies involve much larger numbers of subjects than in Phase 2 and Phase 1, and the subjects will all have the disease or one of the diseases intended to be treated. Two independent, large multicenter studies using the same protocol are ordinarily required for approval of the original indication and often for each new indication as they are sought. There are usually several thousand subjects in total, most often in randomized controlled trials (RCT), aimed at evaluating the efficacy and safety of the test agent in highly-defined and well-controlled settings. In an RCT, patients receive either the drug being tested (the "active" or "test" agent) or the control agent, which may be a commonly used comparator drug or in some cases a placebo. Normally RCTs are double-blinded, which means that neither the patients nor the investigators know which agent, active or control, a given subject is receiving. All human (and animal) testing is approved by institutional review boards (IRBs), usually at each investigative site, although the use of so-called central IRBs with broad jurisdiction are becoming more common, especially for studies by non- university study sites which may not have their own IRB as do universities.

Patients in these RCT trials for regulatory approval are entered into the study based on strict diagnostic criteria, have limited concurrent diseases, are in a tightly controlled age range, use few other medications, are checked for drug taking compliance and followed closely with incentives to not drop out of the study. These circumstances are considerably different than those found in ordinary practice situations. With this in mind, the registration studies are now considered to be evaluating efficacy, the best that might be obtained, in contrast to effectiveness, which is the term applied to the results seen in ordinary practice usage.

Phase 3 trials are the most costly part of a drug development program. Together with Phase 2 trials and depending upon the target indication, e.g., cancer or cardiology, they can easily cost tens of millions of dollars. Phase 3 studies are expected to provide sufficient data to allow the determination of a benefit-to-risk relationship and the creation of the "label." FDA considers any written, printed, or graphic matter that is affixed to, or appears on, a drug or its package to be a label. Labels are required on all drugs involved in interstate commerce or held for sale after shipment or delivery in interstate commerce. The label's content also governs how a drug can be promoted and advertised. Each word of a drug's label has been scrutinized and negotiated by the FDA and the sponsor. The Physician's Desk Reference is largely a collection of drug labels. Labels define the many conditions under which a drug is approved. In addition to the disease(s) for which it is approved, the dosages and the patient populations for which it has been approved are listed as are the side effects.

Using a drug for a disease or a condition, or in a manner not described on the label, gives rise to the phrase "off-label use." Off -label use is very important to the practice of medicine and very common, with up to 50 % of all uses in certain specialties such as oncology being off-label. Since drugs are often not studied in pediatric populations, pediatricians are also forced to use many drugs off-label. Another group often not included in large numbers in the registration studies is the elderly, or over 65- year old group which is frequently the group most likely to use an agent once approved. FDA does encourage inclusion of subjects over 75 years old but there are no requirements for such. At the end of Phase 3 testing, a new drug has usually been used by 1,000–3,000 patients. Given these numbers, it is not surprising that fairly uncommon adverse effects are often not discovered until a drug has been on the market for several years. Overall, about 50 % of approved drugs are ultimately found to have serious adverse effects that were not detected until after FDA approval.

It is interesting to note that some other countries, unlike the United States, have post-marketing safety monitoring done by an organization separate from the organization that gives initial approval to a drug. For example, in the United Kingdom, the drug approval and safety monitoring processes are entirely separate. The safety monitoring unit may order changes in product labeling or the outright withdrawal of a marketed drug. France has a well-developed network of regional pharmacovigilance centers, a national database for practitioners, and a drug safety journal.

The Phase 3 results will, together with the other clinical and preclinical results, be submitted to FDA often as part of an NDA for review for marketing approval. When FDA is criticized for the time needed for agents to reach the market, it is a combination of the time FDA takes to review the ultimate submission as well as the time needed to meet FDA's demanding requirements.

Clinical Study Design and Execution and FDA

Given the importance of human clinical trial results in FDA's approval process, doctors would expect FDA to have a significant interest and expertise in and concern with clinical trial design and good clinical practices. However, physicians might be quite surprised by the broad range of clinical trial design and execution issues in which FDA has offered written advice most commonly in the form of Guidances or Guidance for Industry documents. Although FDA is on record as willing to accept alternative approaches or designs if they satisfy the requirements of the statutes and regulations for proving safety and efficacy, the wide range of issues and specificity of FDA's Guidances on clinical trials execution is illustrative of the complexity of the entire process and of FDA's control of the process.

The following is a large and representative sample of the names of FDA "information sheet guidances" . The titles illustrate in a very educational way the many issues and complexities associated with conducting clinical trials for FDA approval today.

Under the heading of "general information guidance sheets for clinical trials" the following are some of the information sheets available: Charging for Investigation Products; Exception from Informed Consent Requirements for Emergency Research; Acceptance of Foreign Clinical Studies; A Guide to Informed Consent Race and Ethnicity Data in Clinical Trials; Frequently Asked Questions about Institutional Review Boards; Off-Label and Investigational Use of Market Drugs, Biologics and Medical Devices; Payment to Research Subjects; Recruiting Study Subjects; Screening Tests Prior to Study Enrollment; Sponsor-Investigator-IRB Interrelationship; Use of Investigational Products When Subjects Enter a Second Institution; Financial Disclosure by Clinical Investigators; and many others.

Table 10.1 One of many lists of FDA Guidance for Industry documents

Drugs and Biologics Guidance Documents
Available Therapy
Bioavailability and Bioequivalence Testing Samples, Handling and Retention of (PDF – 166 KB)
Clinical Holds Following Clinical Investigator Misconduct, The Use of (PDF – 37 KB)
Clinical Studies Section of Labeling for Human Prescription Drug and Biological Products – Content and Format
Exploratory IND Studies (PDF – 220 KB)
FDA Acceptance of Foreign Clinical Studies Not Conducted Under an IND: Frequently Asked Questions (PDF – 108 KB)
Food-Effect Bioavailability and Fed Bioequivalence Studies (PDF – 166 KB)
Gender Differences in the Clinical Evaluation of Drugs, Guideline for the Study and Evaluation of (PDF – 1.8 MB)
Good Pharmacovigilance Practices and Pharmacoepidemiologic Assessment (PDF – 220 KB)
IND Exemptions for Studies of Lawfully Marketed Drug or Biological Products for the Treatment of Cancer (PDF – 188 KB)
Premarketing Risk Assessment (PDF – 91 KB)
Providing Regulatory Submissions in Electronic Format – Human Pharmaceutical Product Applications and Related Submissions Using the eCTD Specifications
Safety Reporting Requirements for INDs (Investigational New Drug Applications) and BA/BE (Bioavailability/Bioequivalence) Studies (PDF – 227 KB)
Safety Reporting Requirements for INDs and BA/BE Studies- Small Entity Compliance Guide (PDF – 35 KB)
Risk Minimization Action Plans, Development and Use of (PDF – 84 KB)

Also for clinical trials, in addition to the General Information Guidance Sheets above, there are additional lists of guidance sheets under the following large categories: Drugs and Biologics Guidance Documents; Institutional Review Boards (IRBs) and Informed Consent Guidance Documents; Medical Devices Information Sheet Guidance; FDA Operations Information Sheet Guidance; Electronic Data Guidance Documents; and Manufacturing Requirements for Investigational Products Guidance Documents. Under each of these categories are many information sheets. A sense of the detail offered can be seen in the listing in Table 10.1.

Phase 4 Testing

By definition Phase 4 studies are post-marketing studies. An especially important type of Phase 4 study are those which the sponsor promises to conduct as a condition of FDA approval to market. Such "commitment studies" are often required when FDA is approving a drug for a serious unmet medical need in which the clinical studies of the drug used a surrogate endpoint rather than a clinical endpoint. Another category of approvals often associated with the agreement to do mandated post-marketing (Phase 4) studies is the approval of drugs for use in adults which are also likely to be used in a pediatric population but have only been studied in adults. The commitment is then to do post- marketing studies of the drug in a pediatric population with the aim of getting labeling for the pediatric population.

Approvals based on mandated Phase 4 commitment studies have become fairly common and controversial because in most cases the commitment studies have not been done or even started. For example, between 1990 and 1994, 88 new chemical entities were approved, each with one or more Phase 4 commitments. When studied at the end of 1999, only 11 of 88 (13 %) of the mandated Phase 4 studies were complete. Other studies have shown that at most 25 % of the commitment studies have even been started. For 107 drugs approved with a Phase 4 commitment between 1995 and 1999, not one had been completed. Phase 4 studies may confirm the utility and safety of a drug or may find less efficacy, more side effects or other problems. In theory, when a drug is approved based on studies of a surrogate end point, and Phase 4 clinical studies using a clinical endpoint fail to confirm the efficacy or safety seen in the original surrogate based studies, the drug approval should be withdrawn. Although rare, this occurred with the drug Avastin (Bevacizumab), which was approved for metastatic breast cancer using a surrogate endpoint. When the results of two Phase 4 studies conducted by the sponsor failed to find that patients lived any longer or had a better quality of life the indication was removed. Since the drug was also approved for other indications it was not removed from the market.

Phase 4 studies can have many aims. For example, they may be done to generate data for obtaining labeling approval for a new indication, a new dosage or delivery method, long term efficacy or cost benefit. Traditionally known as "marketing studies" and under the control of the marketing or sales divisions of pharmaceutical companies, Phase 4 studies were often criticized for being designed to deliver a favorable outcome to the companies' drugs.

More recently the category of studies known as comparative efficacy studies, which endeavor to compare two or more marketed drugs or treatments using clinical practice conditions for the study rather than FDA study conditions, has led to a new group of post-marketing studies. These clinical trials comparing already marketed agents are considered to be studies of effectiveness rather than efficacy, and while they have little connection to FDA marketing approval they do have considerable potential economic importance. These studies done in the offices of practitioners, using practice conditions such as less stringent disease definition and concomitant use of other drugs, are known as Pragmatic Clinical Trials. In theory, they would have little effect on FDA's view of a drug especially since the drugs usually studied are already marketed, but it will be interesting to see if, in fact, the results of such studies lead in time to FDA actions.

Chapter 11
The New Drug Application (NDA), the Investigative New Drug Exemption (IND) and the General Drug Approval Pathway

The New Drug Application (NDA) is the request to FDA for approval to market the new drug. It is to contain all of the information generated by the sponsor or obtained elsewhere, including the preclinical information such as the chemistry, manufacturing and control information on the active agent, the information usually generated in animal studies on the agent's absorption, distribution, metabolism and excretion, its toxicities and its mechanism of action in the body, and the human or clinical study results (Phases 1–3). The NDA will also contain proposed drug labeling. This information is generated and reported with the aim of giving FDA the basis to decide if: (1) the proposed drug is safe and effective in its intended use(s); (2) the benefits of the proposed drug outweigh the risks; (3) the proposed labeling is suitable; and (4) the proposed drug can be consistently manufactured properly, including its identity, strength, purity and shelf-life.

An NDA for a generic drug will usually not have clinical trials information beyond the blood level studies, and is therefore called an Abbreviated New Drug Application or ANDA. Topicals will need study results using another surrogate or a clinical end-point. Depending upon the complexity, user fees can cost between $500,000 and $5.9 million and do not ensure approval. Provisions are made for a lower fee for new and for smaller companies.

Ordinarily, after completing Phase 3 testing, the sponsor submits the completed New Drug Application to FDA. As indicated, the NDA contains all or summaries of all of the information the sponsor has about the new drug, and on average contains what would be well over 100,000 pages of information. FDA now receives much of this information electronically. As noted elsewhere, the FDA has issued a large number of Guidances covering in great detail the requirements of many elements of the NDA submission.

For some time during the development process, sponsors will have submitted data on their potential drug to FDA for evaluation as part of the process of obtaining permission from FDA to proceed with human testing. The request to permit human testing of the potential drug is called an IND or Investigative New Drug Application Exemption. It is submitted to FDA at the point in drug development when human

© Springer International Publishing Switzerland 2014
W.H. Eaglstein, *The FDA for Doctors*, DOI 10.1007/978-3-319-08362-9_11

testing is thought by the company to be the next step. The IND is an exemption which allows the sponsor to enter their test agent which is not known to be safe (or effective) into interstate commerce for ultimate administration to humans. The IND application includes the non-clinical pharmacology and toxicology information and evidence that the test agent can be made properly. FDA is required to let the sponsor know within 30 days if they may not proceed with the human testing. That is, FDA does not actively approve the human testing.

At various stages in the development process the sponsoring company will meet with FDA members to review the results of their testing under the IND, e.g., an end of Phase 2 testing meeting. At these meetings FDA may conclude that more testing is needed before allowing the next steps, usually more human trials, to proceed. At present this process results in FDA knowing a good deal about the agent before the NDA is finally submitted. Because of the increased number of reviewers and other personnel made available by the Prescription Drug User Fees, FDA's review time for NDAs is one of the shortest in the developed world, averaging about 1 year.

Overall, the pathway for development and FDA approval of a new drug takes in the range of 12–15 years and is estimated to cost between $500 million and $1.5 billion. Dividing the R&D costs of major drug companies by the number of new drugs produced yields figures in the $3–12 billion range, depending upon the company and its number of successful attempts. The major steps in drug development are candidate drug discovery, Preclinical Studies (in vitro and animal), human studies (Phases 1–3) and FDA approval. Should the approval determination be a close call or one with important policy or societal implications, FDA may have recourse to one of the standing or special FDA Advisory Committees. (See Chap. 13). These committees are composed of non-FDA people with special skills who are hired for the committee as special government employees. Their meetings and deliberations are public and their recommendations to FDA are not binding although they are most often followed.

The clinical studies, especially Phase 3, are the most costly portion of the development process, while the FDA review of the approval application, NDA, which takes between 6 months and 2 years, is the least time consuming. Generally, of every 10,000 potential drug candidates, 250 make it through the preclinical phase, 5 of them will reach clinical studies and only 1 will become an approved drug (Fig. 10.1). Of those potential drugs that are evaluated in human trials about 30 % fail due to too many side effects or toxicities, and 50 % fail because they are insufficiently effective. As discussed, FDA approval of most new drugs (and biological drugs) requires two separate large randomized controlled trials, each demonstrating a favorable benefit (efficacy) to risk (toxicity) relationship in the intended indication. By contrast, most devices are cleared by FDA without human trials, and even those devices for which human trials are required may only require one trial. Many OTC drugs are marketed simply by complying with the FDA monograph requirements.

Chapter 12
FDA and Tobacco Products

Much more than most people, doctors realize that health, especially the health of a population, or the public health in general, is dependent on more than health care. Toward that end FDA's role as the regulator of tobacco products is very much consistent with its broad public health mission. However, the regulation of tobacco products represents a somewhat singular or different activity from FDA's general regulatory role in that, unlike the other products FDA regulates, tobacco products are not considered to be safe – their benefits do not outweigh their risks.

Historically, cigarette sales and other tobacco product regulation was done at the state level. While most states ultimately restricted cigarette sales to minors, there were few other state public health efforts related to cigarettes and other tobacco products. In 1965, following a Surgeon General's report that tobacco caused lung cancer, the U.S. Congress passed the Federal Cigarette Labeling and Advertising Act (FCLAA), which required a health warning on all cigarette packs. Shortly thereafter, in 1970, the Public Health Cigarette Smoking Act banned cigarette ads on radio and television and updated the warning on the cigarette package to read: "Warning: The Surgeon General has determined that cigarette smoking is dangerous to your health". Twenty years later, in 1996, FDA issued the "FDA Rule" claiming authority over tobacco use by children, prohibiting non-face-to-face sales of tobacco products and advertising of tobacco products near schools and playgrounds, and other activities which might lead to the use of tobacco products by children. Tobacco companies sued and ultimately the Supreme Court ruled that Congress had not given the FDA authority over tobacco and tobacco marketing. This led to the passage in 2009 of the Family smoking Prevention and Tobacco control Act.

After passage of the Act, which gave FDA the authority to regulate tobacco products, FDA created the Center for Tobacco Products to regulate the manufacture, marketing and distribution of tobacco products to protect public health and to reduce tobacco use. Interestingly and naturally, upon reflection, the law did not give FDA the right to ban the sale of tobacco products, and some tobacco products such as cigars are not regulated by FDA unless therapeutic claims are made for them.

© Springer International Publishing Switzerland 2014
W.H. Eaglstein, *The FDA for Doctors*, DOI 10.1007/978-3-319-08362-9_12

FDA does regulate cigarettes, cigarette tobacco, roll-your-own tobacco, and smoke-less tobacco.

The Center's stated main goals are to prevent Americans—especially youth—from starting to use tobacco, to encourage current users to quit and to decrease the harms of tobacco product use. Using money collected from user fees charged to tobacco manufacturers and importers as authorized by the 2009 Act, FDA is starting a public health information advertising campaign aimed at preventing youths aged 12–17 from starting to smoke. The program, entitled "The Real Cost" campaign, will spend over $100 million in its first year and is based on findings that most smokers start before they are 18 years old. Although the early activities of the FDA at preventing tobacco use, especially among children and youths, has been well accepted, it remains to be seen how well federal efforts to prevent the use of legally sold products will be received over time. Such efforts include more than $273 mil-lion in federal support for 14 Tobacco Centers of Regulatory Science research cen-ters. The centers, most of which are at universities, are to study a variety of subjects including the diversity of tobacco products, reducing addiction, reducing toxicity and carcinogenicity and other adverse health consequences, as well as marketing of tobacco products.

Chapter 13
FDA Advisory Committees

FDA Advisory Committee meetings and their topics are always of great interest to some segment of the regulated community and the associated investment community. Because FDA will often involve an advisory committee for controversial or politically contentious issues such as approval of an OTC drug to induce abortion, or other especially difficult decisions or close calls, advisory committee meetings are often also of great interest to the general public. FDA Advisory Committee meetings are almost always public and although often covered by and reported about in the popular press, the committees themselves, their deliberations and their role or authority are frequently misunderstood. Although FDA advisory committees or panels may be asked to help or offer counsel to FDA over any matter related to FDA's role, including policy and scientific questions, advisory committees attract particularly intense attention when they are asked to advise about an agent's safety and efficacy, and to help in determining the so-called "benefit-to-risk ratio" as part of the final process in determining whether or not to give regulatory approval.

It is important to appreciate that consideration by an advisory committee is not a required or standard part of the deliberative process, that only the FDA, usually at the discretion of one of the division leaders, can bring an issue to an advisory committee and that the decisions or advice of the committee is advisory rather than binding. There are about 50 standing FDA advisory committees and if needed, the agency will appoint an ad hoc committee or add ad hoc members to a standing committee, in order to have the expertise thought to be necessary for the issue at hand. The committees are composed of outside, that is non-FDA, experts and representatives who are not full-time government employees. Rather, the members are appointed as special government employees who are paid for their meeting time and given travel and per diem expenses. The committees meet about four times each year. Each committee has a chair, specialist members, an industry representative, a consumer representative (these are qualified professionals who have connections with relevant consumer advocacy groups or community based organizations) and often a patient representative. Depending upon which areas of FDA the committee is to advise, the specialist members come from fields such as medical

© Springer International Publishing Switzerland 2014
W.H. Eaglstein, *The FDA for Doctors*, DOI 10.1007/978-3-319-08362-9_13

science, pharmacy, nursing, statistics, epidemiology, food safety, toxicology, nutrition, veterinary medicine and so forth.

Members are usually nominated to FDA by organizations and societies although anyone may volunteer or nominate a member. Members must be willing to disclose detailed information about employment, stock holdings, research grants and other information related to potential financial and other conflicts. Candidates with too many potential conflicts may not be selected as their ability to participate fully might be too limited. Membership and the degree of participation by advisory committee members has been a difficult and sometimes contentious issue. Often those most expert, whose insights and advice would be most valuable to FDA, are also the most potentially conflicted. Traditionally FDA has been able to grant conflict of interest waivers allowing, under defined circumstances, participation of individuals whose services are considered to be valuable enough to outweigh the potential conflict of interest. At one time the number of people serving based on such waivers was limited or capped. At present, based somewhat on studies of the effect of conflicts on committee activities, the cap is no longer applied. Participation, or the term of service, is usually 4 years and requires a significant commitment of effort and time. The committee members individually review written information and questions sent to them by FDA before their formal, public meetings, which are usually in the Washington, D.C. area. The meetings are open to the public and members of the public may not only attend but may also speak to the committee, although to do so usually requires making arrangements in advance of the meeting.

At the FDA Advisory Committee meetings, the members hear directly from the sponsor when, as is most often the case, the decision will bear on an approval, from the FDA and from other interested parties such as patient organizations. The panels are convened to answer specific questions posed by FDA about the issue or application. FDA's questions to the committee which are written and are part of the public record, often include the broad issue of whether the sponsor has demonstrated safety and efficacy for the intended drug or agents use. With regard to approvals, the committees most often reach conclusions that back or support approval for drugs, devices, biologics and other agents. In one recent and typical year, advisory panels backed approval for 76 % of new drugs and 82 % of new medical devices, and although not required to do so, FDA most often follows the advice from its advisory committees. Because approvals carry so much importance to the financial well-being of the sponsors and because panels are asked for their opinions on the most difficult situations, the panels' answers or conclusions are almost always reported in the popular press, leading patients and others to the misunderstanding that a new agent has been approved and is on the market. Advisory Committee answers will also often lead to changes, sometimes dramatic, in a stock's price in anticipation of FDA approval or disapproval as suggested by the committee.

Chapter 14
FDA, Labels and Labeling for Medical Products

FDA-approved labels of prescription drugs and biologicals are very important to doctors and are written primarily to help doctors use the agent safely and effectively. Recognizing that labeling should also help patients, in 1970 FDA first required the now commonly used Patient Package Insert to help patients better understand the benefits and risks of prescription drugs. Prescription drug labels are also referred to as the prescribing information. Package inserts, package circulars and other associated written materials are all considered part of the product label. The information on the label will also guide and limit advertising and promotion. Broadly, the label is a compilation of information about the product which, while written by the manufacturer, must be approved by FDA. The label is, of course, based on the information submitted to FDA in the new drug application, biological license application or other relevant application. FDA's analysis of and conclusions about this information determine what gets printed on the label.

Doctors may not realize that prescription drug labels must follow a specific format known as the SPL, or structured product label, format. The SPL format has been developed by industry sponsors of prescription and OTC drugs, FDA, product distributors and a group involved in international informatics and labeling. Since FDA's requirement for SPL is being phased in and was not even required for non-prescription drugs until 2009, not all agents have an SPL.

Briefly, the SPL format has three large sections: the highlights section, the table of contents and the full prescribing information. The type of information which must be on the label, for example, the listing of other names for the agent, and the date of its approval by FDA is mandated, as is the order of the sections. Of special note is the section physicians refer to as the Black Box, which FDA calls the Boxed Warning section. This information, circumscribed by a dramatic wide and deep colored black line, is consider very essential and contains warnings which are often so alarming as to reduce the frequency of prescribing by physicians, or cause doctors to discuss the situation with their patients with the result that patients do not take the drug. Black boxed warnings are often added to the label after approval and considerable time on the market, when new toxicities or drug-related issues are learned

© Springer International Publishing Switzerland 2014
W.H. Eaglstein, *The FDA for Doctors*, DOI 10.1007/978-3-319-08362-9_14

about. As can be imagined, the Boxed Warning section is often the subject of intense negotiation between the company selling the drug and FDA. Although Boxed Warnings appear in the highlights section of the label, by regulation the information in the box in the highlights section is limited to 20 lines. Therefore, the complete warning may only be found in the Full Prescribing Information section.

The guidelines for device labeling, while similar to those for drug labeling are separate. For devices, FDA considers the label as any written or graphic material on the immediate container of the item and any articles, posters, tags, pamphlets, circulars, booklets, brochures, instruction books, direction sheets, fillers and so forth that are offered with the device. However, the information on device labels is not presented in the SPL format. Other differences between drug and device labeling requirements include device provisions, such as requiring that the manufacturer or distributor provide labeling adequate to use the device for a use which was not originally intended. For example, a manufacturer of dental X-ray equipment who is routinely selling his product to podiatrists would be required to provide labeling for its podiatric use. Most recently FDA has started a program, beginning with Class 3 devices (those with the greatest potential to be harmful), requiring that each device carry a unique device identifier or UDI. This program is aimed at improving safety by allowing problems to be associated with a specific device, and making it possible, for example, to rapidly recall defective implanted heart valves. As is the case for drugs, most if not all advertising is governed by the approved label and may be considered to be labeling.

Of course, it has always been recognized that labeling for non-prescription or OTC drugs is aimed at the consumer. As noted in the chapter on non-prescription drugs, FDA approval is dependent upon users being able to understand how to use the drug, in addition to being able to self-diagnose the need for the drug, and for a very high level of drug safety. Based on rules finalized by FDA in 1999, over 100,000 OTC products are now labeled in a consistent way with all of the information listed and arranged in the same order. Briefly, the information required and the order is to be: active ingredient (including the amount of active ingredient per unit); uses; warnings; inactive ingredients; purpose and directions. The label is also required to include the lot or batch number, the expiration date, name and address of the manufacturer, packer or distributor, quantity of contents, and what to do if an overdose occurs. The label must also describe how to open the package, especially when tamper-proof containers are required. Although FDA controls the labeling of OTC drugs, which includes the written material on the container and any written information accompanying the package, the Federal Trade Commission and not the FDA regulates advertising of OTC drugs. While FDA-approved labeling guides prescription drug advertising, and even though the FTC Act requires that all advertising be truthful and non-deceptive, that advertisers have evidence to back up their claims and that advertisements not be unfair, the implementation of these requirements for OTC drugs leads to considerable variance between advertisements for prescription drugs and OTC drugs. Doctors will find it helpful to realize that this gap may exist or occur between the information their patients read on OTC labels and the information they find in advertisements.

Chapter 15
FDA and Product Names

Many doctors might be surprised to learn that FDA must approve a drug's proprietary or brand name before the drug is allowed on the market. The requirement for pre-market approval of the brand name is primarily to avoid confusion and errors because of drugs having names which are very similar. Medication errors are actually very common and estimated to lead to death in 7,000 people annually. Obviously, having similarly named drugs on the market can cause medication errors, and FDA data suggests that nearly 13 % of medication errors are related to confusion over medication names. Studies show that more than 30 % of all handwritten prescriptions contained a mistake of some type that required deciphering and correcting by a pharmacist. (Even though FDA has programs to prevent the marketing of drug names which might be confused with another drug, many, for example Adderal and Inderal or Noroxin and Neurontin, are nevertheless on the market. The Institute for Safe Medication Practices List of Confused Drug Names has several hundred examples!!)

With the goal of not approving drug names that might lead to confusion, the CDER division of Medication Error Prevention and Analysis compares proposed brand names, including the names of generic drugs, to the names of already approved drugs and to proposed names for drugs being reviewed for approval. The FDA evaluation is fairly thorough as the proposed names are compared for their spelling, their appearance when written (a variety of handwriters are compared) and for pronunciation when spoken. The FDA review and approval must be obtained before the US Patent and Trade Mark Office issues the proprietary name. In the United States there are over 30,000 separate proprietary or brand named drugs on the market. As doctors and much of the public realize, proprietary drugs also have generic names and these do not need FDA approval, while the brand names of generic drugs do need approval. Drugs, or at least their active agents, also have a chemical name which again does not need FDA approval.

As noted, name reviews are very formal and involve generating lists of names which might be confused with the proposed name and testing to compare the chance that the names might be confused either in handwritten, printed or spoken communication. In addition to the review to ensure safety, the Division of Drug Marketing, Advertising, and

© Springer International Publishing Switzerland 2014
W.H. Eaglstein, *The FDA for Doctors*, DOI 10.1007/978-3-319-08362-9_15

Communications conducts a so called Promotional Review. This review aims to determine if the proposed proprietary name misleadingly implies singular efficacy, suggests unproved superiority to other products, suggests a broader indication than is labeled or minimizes risks. So-called fanciful names are also rejected. FDA may even reject brand names already given formal trademark registration from the U.S. Patent and Trademark Office. Overall, each year FDA reviews over 500 proposed new proprietary drug names and rejects about one-third of them. In addition, to prevent post-approval confusion, FDA reviews about 1,400 medication error reports per month and can demand changes to brand names or product labeling based on reports of confusion in the marketplace. Since pharmaceutical and other companies spend considerable sums in selecting a product name (often between $200,000 and $300,000 dollars for one drug name), in getting a trademark, and even on the early printing of materials for ultimate marketing use, the rejection of a name by FDA can result in loss of such expenditures in addition to the loss of revenue occasioned by the postponement of the launch or initial marketing date.

Interestingly and importantly, for both doctors and patients, FDA does not control use of the brand name on many OTC products. Although the ingredients, including the active agent, are listed on all OTC products, the same brand or proprietary name may be used on several products that actually contain different active ingredients. For example, four OTC products use the trade name Mylanta: Mylanta AR®, Mylanta® Cherry Creme Liquid, Mylanta® Gas Relief and Mylanta® Double Strength. The active ingredients are, respectively: famotidine; aluminum hydroxide, magnesium hydroxide and simethicone; simethicone; and calcium carbonate and magnesium hydroxide. Allegra® has four different dosages, each for a different age group, but all carry the name Allegra®. Similarly, Benadryl® is used in the name of several different OTC products. Although careful inspection can determine the differences between these products, doctors all know of occasions when patients have inadvertently been using the wrong OTC product.

With regard to device names, while FDA has the same responsibility to prevent names which might produce medical error, names that imply an untrue level of efficacy and/or names which mislead regarding safety or superiority, its review of device names is not at the same level of scrutiny as that for drugs. This is because unlike pills and other medications, devices are most often clearly distinct one from another. For example, the surgical team implanting a heart valve will not mistake a bone screw for the valve regardless of the similarity of their names. That being said, FDA does from time to time demand that a device implement a name change based on FDA's mandate to prevent "mislabeling".

Chapter 16
FDA and Promotion and Advertising

Companies spend more on marketing/advertising than on research. Of the estimated $57 billion spent in the U.S., 50 % is spent on free samples, 30 % on detailing physicians and hospitals and 15 % on medical journal and direct-to-consumer advertising. While the Food Drug and Cosmetic Act does not authorize regulation of the practice of medicine by FDA, it does call for FDA to regulate the promotion of prescription drugs (OTC drug promotion is regulated by the Federal Trade Commission) and certain devices. In regulating drug promotion, FDA requires that advertising be based on substantial evidence or clinical experience (which has come to mean on the labeled information), be truthful and not misleading and present a "fair balance" of risk and benefit. All promotional materials and efforts must be consistent with the FDA approved labeling.

For doctors, labeling is an especially key issue. FDA considers promotion and promotional materials to be unlawful if they promote unlabeled, that is unapproved, uses of these products. For example, promoting a use for a drug or device which is not described as indicated on the drug or device label, a so called off-label use, is illegal. Even promotion or description of new dosing schedules or dosing amounts is illegal. Such off-label recommendations or uses are, for dramatic effect, sometimes called illegal or unapproved uses rather than the more balanced phrases, off-label, unlabeled or extra-label.

It is important to remember that it is not the off-label use recommended or prescribed by physicians that is illegal. It is the promotion of such by companies that has been considered illegal. Of course, based on articles, textbooks, lectures and other such information, physicians frequently use drugs and devices off-label. In some instances and in some fields the off-label usage may far exceed the labeled usage. For example, oncologists use many agents in series and combinations which have never been approved on the labels. Similarly, pediatricians use drugs with children that have never been approved for children. To stimulate companies to study and apply for labeling for pediatric uses, FDA has offered a period of exclusivity to companies which do formal studies on the use of agents in pediatric patients.

© Springer International Publishing Switzerland 2014
W.H. Eaglstein, *The FDA for Doctors*, DOI 10.1007/978-3-319-08362-9_16

Despite the many situations in which physicians use agents off-label, many physicians, especially generalists, are frequently reluctant to offer off-label therapies. Understanding the FDA's strict requirement that promotion adhere to the label, we can appreciate the significance of a recent United States appellate court ruling that when speaking to physicians, pharmaceutical representatives have the right to discuss off-label uses of a drug. The court ruled that this was within the representatives' right to free speech, just as it would be for a doctor or anyone else discussing off-label information and uses. Of course, such discussion must be based on true information and not be false or misleading.

The "fair balance" requirement for advertising is especially important for both doctors and the public. Fair balance does not require that risks and benefits of a drug receive equal space and word size in print or time in broadcast promotions. Rather, fair balance requires that the content and presentation of a drug's most important risks be reasonably similar to the content and presentation of its benefits. Physicians and the public are encouraged by FDA to report inequities to The Bad Ad Program which is administered by the agency's Office of Prescription Drug Promotion (OPDP) in the Center for Drug Evaluation and Research.

Interestingly, the U.S. and New Zealand are the only countries in the world which allow direct to consumer advertising (DTCA) of prescription pharmaceuticals. FDA only permitted such advertising starting in the mid-1990s. The effect of DTCA as seen in print and on television and radio is of great interest and consequence to patients, physicians and FDA. In 2004 FDA reported the results of their survey of 500 doctors, which was part of FDA's attempt to understand the effect of DTCA on the patient- doctor relationship, patients, doctors and the practice of medicine. The doctor survey found that: (1) Most physicians believed patients who had seen DTC ads asked thoughtful questions, were more involved with their care and were more aware of possible treatments; (2) While only 8 % of doctors felt very pressured to prescribe the drug discussed in the DTC ads, 75 % of doctors felt the DTC ads made patients think the drug worked better than it did, 65 % of doctors felt the ads confused their patients and only 40 % felt their patients understood the possible risks of the advertised drugs. This doctor survey was preceded by two surveys of the public and in conjunction with advertising surveys, phone interviews and reports, all of which, in aggregate, seem to have satisfied FDA that the DTC program should be continued.

Because drug advertising to physicians (and to the public) have so much potential for affecting the physician-patient interaction and for misunderstanding, it is worthwhile discussing the FDA's regulations and policies in considerable detail. It is important to realize that FDA only receives advertisements from the companies when they are released. That is, companies must submit their advertisements to FDA only when they are first released to the public. FDA does not review advertisements, whether to physicians or the public, before they are released. Companies may query FDA before releasing an ad but that is not required. This approach means that the public or physicians may see advertisements which break the law or violate FDA regulations before FDA is able to request that the advertisements be withdrawn. Also, FDA has no control over the amount of money companies may spend promoting drugs and has no special authority over advertising for agents which might be especially dangerous or damaging.

Although FDA cannot control the exact type of words used in ads, e.g., windpipe vs trachea, all ads must give at least one approved use for the drug, its generic name and all or the most important risks. An exception to this rule is the so-called reminder ad, which gives the drug's name but not its use. The assumption behind reminder ads is that the audience knows what the drug is for and does not need to be told. A reminder ad does not contain risk information about the drug because the ad does not discuss the condition treated or how well the drug works. Although some critics believe they should, ads are not required to include information on how a drug works, the likelihood or speed with which it might work or if there is a generic version of the drug.

Doctors are particularly familiar with the package insert which is also known as prescribing information, product information, product labeling or the PI. It is the most complete information about a prescription drug, containing technical information such as the chemistry of the drug, its use in specific conditions and complete detail about side effects. The prescribing information is a key part of FDA's final drug approval and it is written for doctors rather than for the public. When promotions and advertising fail to follow these and other FDA regulations, FDA generally asks the drug company to remove the unlawful ad. If there is a possibility of a serious public health problem because of the ad, the company may be asked to publish a corrective ad. Additional actions can include seizure of the drug from supply lines and bringing criminal charges.

Because of its public impact, relative "newness" and its potential to affect doctor-patient interactions, direct to consumer advertising has evoked a wide array of reactions among physicians and public health investigators as well as the public. In fact, as noted above, a surprisingly large body of research on the effects of DTCA has been developed. Most broadly, critics and proponents of DTCA differ as to whether it improves public health by leading to more treatment and better compliance for patients who have been under-treated, or whether it is a threat to public health since it leads to unnecessary treatment and associated increased risks and resource utilization.

FDA's rationale for allowing DTCA is that, in contrast to paradigms of the past in which patients were passive recipients of care dispensed by all knowing physicians, patients are now active participants in their care. The many issues occasioned by DTCA may be placed into a number of categories, such as the educational value of DTCA; its ability to produce a better quality of care and patient-doctor interaction; its promotion of better patient adherence; its promotion of over-diagnosis and medicalization of nonmedical problems; and the promotion of questionable prescribing habits. Studies of these issues have largely produced mixed results with few clear answers.

Critics of the current DTCA programs have asked for many changes, such as requiring that the ads include information on: (1) lifestyle changes which patients might undertake in addition to drugs; (2) the cost of the drugs being advertised; (3) alternative drugs which might be used; (4) more risk information presented in a more balanced fashion; (5) more quantitative information about likely benefits and risks; and (6) use of eighth grade-level language. Interestingly, studies of doctor's impressions of the effects of DTCA are as mixed as are all of the other study results. Some critics have compared our country's experience with DTCA to a large uncontrolled public health study.

Adding to the experiment is FDA's own venture into advertising. In 2009 Congress passed the Family Smoking Prevention and Tobacco Control Act which gave FDA the authority to regulate tobacco products, based on the idea that tobacco use is the leading cause of preventable health problems. Using the new powers granted under this act, FDA, through its Center for Tobacco Products, is spending in the first year of the campaign $115 million on television and other forms of advertisement as part of its first national public education campaign to prevent youth tobacco use and to reduce the number of kids ages 12–17 who become regular smokers. The advertising is aimed at people aged 12–17 years old because 90 % of adult smokers are known to have started smoking before age 18. Advertising by FDA is a fairly new and largely unregulated and unproven public health effort. It remains to be seen if advertising by the federal government against the purchase of a legally sold product will be extended to adults and how it will be received.

Chapter 17
Off-Label Use

Off-label use of drugs and other agents can be very anxiety-producing for doctors because of concerns related to potential malpractice suits. Until quite recently, once an agent was approved it could only be marketed/promoted by the pharmaceutical company for the use or disease indication (intended indication) and in the manner described on the approved written instructions and information or drug label. Uses of the drug to treat other conditions or uses in manners not described on the label are called "off-label" uses. Sometimes, off-label uses are called "unapproved uses" or even "illegal uses". Using the words "illegal" and "unapproved" is most often intended to convey a characterization which is inappropriate but it does occur, especially when condemning certain medical practices or as part of a malpractice suit attempt. Because the FDA-approved written instructions and information ("label") are based on information available from the studies submitted in order to obtain marketing approval, the label often ends up being quite narrow compared to a drug's actual use as determined in practice and by studies not used for FDA approval or label changes. For example, after approval and broad availability and use of a drug, new indications are found based on serendipitous observations and empiric evidence. There is a widening of the criteria for use even for patients who have the labeled indication, because, for example, the diagnostic criteria for the labeled indication are loosened, or combinations of the drug with other agents become the standard of care.

Off-label treatment is fully legal and is very common. For example, many pediatric treatments are off-label because few drugs have been developed for and studied in children. Even using an unlabeled dose, or treating patients older or younger than the age indicated on the label, or using a dosing frequency which is not described makes the drug's use off-label. Many of the combination chemotherapy regimens used in oncology have not been approved by FDA, are not described on the label and are considered off-label. For reasons such as these, large numbers of cancer chemotherapy drugs and drugs used in children are in fact used off-label. To overcome this problem in children, FDA has offered an additional 6 months of market exclusivity to sponsors for studying and obtaining labeling for pediatric use.

© Springer International Publishing Switzerland 2014
W.H. Eaglstein, *The FDA for Doctors*, DOI 10.1007/978-3-319-08362-9_17

Congress has been clear in its intent that the FDA should not interfere with the practice of medicine. As long as the physician is prescribing an approved drug for an off-label use to help the well- being of an individual patient, and has a reasonable scientific basis for expecting success. The off-label use is within the context of the practice of medicine. Such therapy may be referred to as "innovative therapy". It should be noted that sponsors do seek label changes from time to time, most often to add a new indication or to broaden the intended treatment populations and toward that end, new study results are submitted to FDA for approval. As noted earlier, until recently it was illegal for companies to promote the off-label use of a drug. However it is now legal to send physicians studies and other information on off-label drug use if such information is requested by the physician and the request is spontaneous, that is, not stimulated by the company. It has also been ruled that pharmaceutical representatives have the right to discuss off-label use as part of their constitutionally guaranteed right of free speech.

The status of off-labeled drug usage in the eyes of insurance companies is quite variable. Obviously insurance payment for drugs is often crucial to their off-label use. However, as doctors are usually aware, insurance companies often resist paying for expensive drugs if they are to be used off-label. Physicians frequently have to jump through a number of bureaucratic hoops to enable patients to have coverage for their medicine costs when their use is off-label. Finally it should be noted that off-label use can occur with both prescription and non-prescription (OTC) drugs although the former is more often contentious.

Chapter 18
Additional Drug Approval Pathways and Expanded Access (Treatment INDs); and Personal Importation of Unapproved Drugs

For drugs and biologics, in addition to the normal approval pathways already described, there are several other pathways or methodologies for making drugs available that are offered by FDA. They are all aimed at speeding the development and availability of drugs to prevent or treat serious diseases. In large measure these pathways were developed and approved due to pressures placed on the government and especially on the FDA by the AIDS community for speedier development and approval of drugs to treat AIDS. The 1990 protests by AIDS activists in front of the FDA's headquarters was among the most visible efforts. Although other communities, such as the cancer community, had similar issues, the AIDS community consisted of younger and better organized sufferers and supporters, who were better able to make their case politically and ultimately successfully.

To use these additional and "new" approval pathways, the drug being developed must be either the first to prevent or to treat the disease, or a drug which has significant advantages over the existing treatments. That is, the potential drug must be aimed at filling an "unmet medical need" and the disease must be "serious". Serious disease usually means a lethal disease, a disease which adversely affects day to day living, or a disease which if left untreated will become serious.

The pathways or approaches available for potential drugs meeting these unmet medical needs and serious criteria are known as Priority Review, Accelerated Approval, Fast Track and Breakthrough Therapy (Table 18.1) Because these names are all fanciful and all tend to advertise an inflated sense of speediness they are easily confused, difficult to understand and would probably not meet FDA's standards for a proprietary drug name. Accelerated Approval, Priority Review and Fast Track have been available for some time, while Breakthrough Therapy is more recent and includes all of the benefits of the Fast Track designation plus others.

The key feature of the Accelerated Approval pathway or designation is that FDA agrees to base its regulatory decision on a patient outcome that is a surrogate or substitute outcome rather than on the primary clinical outcome. A surrogate endpoint is a measure rather than a clinical outcome or clinical benefit, such as enhanced survival, improved function or better feeling. For example, if the clinical outcome is

© Springer International Publishing Switzerland 2014
W.H. Eaglstein, *The FDA for Doctors*, DOI 10.1007/978-3-319-08362-9_18

Table 18.1 Approval pathways for serious disease and unmet medical need

Pathway name	Surrogate end point	Fast review	Extra FDA guidance
Accelerated approval	×		
Priority review		×	
Fast track	×	×	
Break through	×	×	×

stroke the surrogate endpoint might be to measure blood pressure. While prevention of stroke might take many years to prove, studies of blood pressure reduction can be done relatively rapidly. Similarly, reduction in a tumor size, a measure, would be more rapid than studies to show a reduction in death from cancers, and a reduction in blood cholesterol levels (a measure) is faster (and less expensive) than studies of reduced myocardial infarction. AIDS drugs were approved on the measured number of CD4 cells (and now HIV-1 viral load) rather than survival.

It is important to remember that to qualify for Accelerated Approval and the other faster pathways, the drug must be for a serious disease and must satisfy an unmet medical need, which would include having far fewer side effects than the available therapy. Once approved for marketing on the basis of a surrogate endpoint, FDA requires that additional studies, so called post-marketing or phase 4 studies, be done by the sponsor to document that the drug actually produces the clinical outcome thought to be indicated by the surrogate endpoint. For example, the drug should reduce deaths from tumors which the drug was shown to shrink. Should phase 4 studies fail to document the clinical benefit, the drug is to be taken off the market. Unfortunately, companies frequently do not do the phase 4 studies to which they have committed.

The key element in the Priority Review designation is FDA's commitment to review the drug or biological application within 6 months, as compared to the 10 or more months which is standard. Agents which offer significant improvements in the safety or effectiveness of the treatment, diagnosis, or prevention of serious conditions when compared to standard treatments are given Priority Review status. Actually, FDA reviews each new IND application for its eligibility for Priority Review. Although valuable, a faster review does not change the many years needed by the sponsor to develop the data needed to apply for approval.

Fast Track designation, which must be requested by the sponsor, provides the benefits of Accelerated Approval and Priority Review. That is, the Fast Track designation provides: the surrogate endpoint; the 6 month review time; valuable assistance from FDA such as frequent meetings, frequent correspondence to ensure appropriate clinical study design, surrogate endpoints and data collection as needed to support drug approval; and a so-called Rolling Review, which allows the sponsor to submit completed sections of its application to FDA for review as each section is developed rather than having to wait for completion of the entire application as is normally required.

Breakthrough Therapy offers all of the benefits of Fast Track (fast and rolling review and surrogate endpoints) plus the involvement of senior FDA managers and early intensive guidance. Breakthrough Therapy designation has been developed in response to the development of drugs, often biological drugs, which target specific molecular pathways known to be operative in the recipient population such that early dramatic clinical effects are obtainable. As such, the key to obtaining Breakthrough Therapy designation is obtaining data early in the clinical development phase indicating that the drug may demonstrate substantial improvement over existing therapies on one or more clinically significant endpoints. The sponsor may request or FDA may suggest this designation, but in either case the evaluation is to be made early, before the end of the phase 2 meeting with FDA.

Access to investigational or unapproved drugs for treatment outside of a clinical study is often referred to by the phrase "compassionate treatment" or discussed under the topic of "expanded access". However, such use is considered by FDA to be a "treatment use" and is allowed by an exemption called a "Single Use Treatment IND" if it is for a single person or a "Treatment IND" if it is for use by a group of people. These treatment uses are considered investigational because data on safety and efficacy are kept and reported.

Treatment INDs are usually thought of and may only be approved after there is some indication that a drug may be effective and without catastrophic side effects. This means that the drug is probably under study in clinical trials. Usually a physician will apply to FDA for the treatment IND. A number of elements are need for FDA to approve: the person or persons being treated must have a serious or immediately life threatening condition such as terminal AIDS or a viral encephalitis; there should not be alternative treatments available for the person; and the sponsor should be pursuing approval to market, which means clinical trials are underway or completed and Investigative Review Board (IRB) approval, including an informed consent, must be obtained, or in the case of an emergency the applicant must assure FDA that approval will be sought. Of course, to actually treat with the unapproved drug, even when FDA approval is obtained, the drug must be available, which may not always be the case. The drug sponsor may not have sufficient drug manufactured or may be unwilling to provide the drug for other reasons including cost. FDA does allow companies to charge for the cost of drugs provided under a Treatment IND but insurance companies rarely agree to pay for experimental or unapproved drugs.

As is the case for many FDA policies, those dealing with the importation of unapproved drugs for personal use are somewhat complex. Most often these complexities are a result of trying to make policy which can be applied to a large population with so many variables at play. Shipping unapproved drugs between states is illegal and that includes importing them from other countries. Illegally imported drugs are often seized and the parties involved are subject to legal penalties. However, FDA recognizes that there are many circumstances under which FDA should not exercise its prohibitory power over the importation of non-FDA approved drugs. For example, foreign visitors or even citizens who need to complete a course of therapy with a drug originally obtained and started outside of the United States, might reasonably be allowed to import the drug in order to finish their treatments. In fact, FDA's guidance to its employees suggests regulatory forbearance in order to avoid overburdening the Agency. The general conditions outlined as guidances but not as mandates for regulatory discretion or tolerance of importation for personal use, apply to citizens as well as non-citizens. The circumstances when FDA will tolerate drug importation for personal use include when the drug is for a serious disease for which there is no approved treatment available in the U.S. and the unapproved drug is not considered to pose an unreasonable risk (a level of paternalism not uncommon in FDA "thinking", which is often criticized). Additionally, there is to be no intent to commercialize or promote the unapproved drug to others. The person for whom the drug is intended must testify in writing that the drug is for personal use and the U.S. licensed doctor caring for the person receiving the drug must be identified. Generally no more than 3 months' worth of drug is allowed to be imported at one time. Obviously, by taking responsibility for and by implication assuring FDA that the unapproved drug is not thought to be associated with unreasonable risk, physicians play a key role in helping patients obtain FDA's approval for the importation and use of unapproved drugs. Equally obvious is the fact that such regulatory forbearance is not given to bring into the U.S. versions of FDA approved drugs which are attractively priced but which have not been manufactured at sites approved by FDA or labeled with FDA oversight.

Chapter 19
FDA Exclusivity and Patents

Patents, formally known as intellectual property or IP, are a government-granted monopoly or ownership of an idea (hence intellectual property). The ownership is granted for a certain period of time, known as the patent life. Patents are offered in order to guarantee that the information will be made public and ultimately useful to all. This is in contrast to a trade secret, such as the formula for Coca-Cola, which remains generally unknown after being on the market in one form or another since the 1880s. Patents are vital to drug developers because they offer some assurance that the cost to develop innovative agents can be recouped and a profit made. When drugs are protected by IP their prices are usually high, falling by an average of 80 % within 2 years after the generic versions are ultimately marketed. A dramatic example of this is anti-HIV drugs. Patented anti-HIV drugs in the year 2000 cost about $10,000/year per person, while 13 years later generic versions of the same drugs cost about $150/year.

Even though patents are critical to those willing to take the risk to develop drugs and other medical products, patents are not issued by FDA but rather are issued by the US Patent and Trademark Office (PTO). As regards drug development, patents may be granted for the method of using the drug (use patent), the manufacturing process (process patent), the formulation (formulation patent) or for the drug chemical itself (a composition-of-matter or product patent) (Table 19.1). While each of these patent types has its advantages, the composition-of-matter patent is considered strongest. Patents offer ownership exclusivity for 20 years, but since meeting FDA's marketing requirements may consume many of these 20 years, the effective protection or the period during which a product is protected from competition and may be sold or marketed is usually much less than 20 years. Drug developers often develop a group or family of patents around a drug, for example, one patent for the initial chemical composition of the active agent and then additional patents for the salt, ester and other forms of the active agent. Among the aims of creating this patent family, especially when the second and subsequent patents are sought some time after the initial patent, is extension of the length or term of total patent protection time. This practice is sometimes called "ever greening" or life-cycle management.

© Springer International Publishing Switzerland 2014

W.H. Eaglstein, *The FDA for Doctors*, DOI 10.1007/978-3-319-08362-9_19

Table 19.1 Patents are
important to drug
development

Patents
Government granted idea ownership (intellectual property)
Given by U.S. Patent and Trademark Office
Common pharmaceutical types
Composition-of-matter- active agent
Process – method of production
Method-of-use – use to treat a disease

Some critics believe that extending the patent-protected life of drugs in this manner, especially when applied to poor countries, unfairly keeps prices high and also misallocates resources away from true innovation.

Although not able to offer patent protection, FDA is able to issue marketing exclusivity, often referred to as Exclusivity, to certain categories of products under its jurisdiction. That is, for a certain period of time FDA will not approve a competing product or, if the product is already on the market, will not approve a label change, thereby providing, at least in the United States, a period of market exclusivity. There are various types of exclusivity, and depending upon the type exclusivity may run concurrently or independently of the patent tenure. FDA offers exclusivity either as a reward for risk taking, innovation and creativity or as an inducement to other behaviors FDA wishes to foster. Examples of the latter include the orphan drug exclusivity and the pediatric exclusivity.

Orphan drugs are drugs which are developed to treat diseases which affect small numbers of people (by definition in the U.S 200,000 individuals). Such drugs are considered to be orphans since companies have traditionally not been willing to undertake their development because of the small potential market. However, this has changed recently because companies have been given exclusivity for their orphan drugs and because the orphan diseases are often lethal or totally debilitating. Patients and their insurance companies have been willing to pay thousands of dollars per year for the drugs, which treat illnesses which are often chronic. As a result, orphan drugs have become large revenue generators. As one part of the package of inducements/rewards for development of an orphan drug, FDA offers 7 years of marketing exclusivity.

Because historically few drugs were studied in children, FDA offered 6 months of exclusivity to companies which study their drug in the pediatric population. The pediatric exclusivity applies an additional 6 months to either the patent term or another exclusivity. Interestingly, pediatric exclusivity is granted to all forms of the drug entity; for example oral, iv and topical, based on the study of any one form, and the exclusivity is independent of actually obtaining a labeling change.

In the "rewards" category, FDA gives a 5-year exclusivity for development of a new chemical entity, a so- called NCE exclusivity, and 3 years for doing clinical studies and obtaining clinical data for a new use of an already marketed drug. These so called new drug product exclusivities are automatically afforded drugs which qualify, in contrast to other forms of FDA exclusivity for which companies need to apply.

In addition to the two new product exclusivities, the pediatric exclusivity and the orphan drug exclusivity, FDA affords a patent challenge or generic drug exclusivity, most often called the 180-day exclusivity. The 180-day exclusivity is offered to encourage and reward development of generic drugs. The fact that 180 days, approximately 6 months, of exclusivity is so desirable is testimony to the profitability of producing a generic drug, at least until many generics of that agent are on the market. The 180-day exclusivity is given to the first generic to qualify. During the 180 days after the initial generic receives its approval, approvals for the same generic drug produced by another company are withheld. The 180-day exclusivity is associated with a great deal of controversy and litigation. Much of the controversy is related to situations in which the generic applicant, in order to be able to obtain approval and market a generic version of a patented drug, asserts that the patent of the pioneer drug was invalid. Most often this is one of the life-cycle extending sorts of patents. The other area of controversy relates to the situation in which FDA approved the first generic and gives the 180 day exclusivity but the company, rather than offering the generic on the market, takes payment from the company with the pioneer drug as compensation for not marketing the generic. The result is that the public continues to pay high prices rather than having the opportunity to pay a reduced price for a generic version of the drug.

Finally, FDA cooperates with the Patent and Trademark Office in affording the developing company a patent term restoration or patent term extension as compensation for the patent time lost in meeting FDA approval requirements. The patent term restoration or extension cannot be for more than 5 years, and FDA's role is to advise the patent office of the regulatory circumstances to be considered in offering the restoration.

Overall, FDA exclusivity has significant financial implications and allows FDA to guide companies toward actions deemed important to the public. These exclusivities also result in considerable rule- making and litigation and can have unintended consequences. Although not given directly by FDA, restoration of the patent time is also important is stimulating companies to undertake development of new drugs.

Chapter 20
Adverse Event Reporting, Pharmacovigilance and FDA

In the United States, the FDA is responsible for drug safety or pharmacovigilance. Although the word pharmacovigilance, combining the Greek word for drugs and the Latin word for watch, might suggest it relates only to drug safety, pharmacovigilance usually also applies to medical device safety. Pharmacovigilance is not a word often encountered in the medical literature most doctors read. The World Health Organization defines pharmacovigilance as: "The science and activities relating to the detection, assessment, understanding and prevention of adverse effects or any drug-related problem." Generally, pharmacovigilance has been taken up more formally in other countries than it has been in the United States. Because the FDA is the agency which approves drugs and devices, judging them to be sufficiently safe and effective and allowing them to be marketed, critics often point out that it is inappropriate for FDA to also be in charge of monitoring and assuring ultimate safety once marketed since FDA might be reluctant to conclude their initial judgment was incorrect. In some countries the approval and the marketing surveillance activities are handled by separate agencies.

Although FDA is charged with monitoring both drug and device safety, it is important to recognize that drug and device adverse events are considerably different and require different methods of classification, reporting and management. In the drug area, there is usually little need to be concerned with how to administer the product. For example, it is obvious to us how to swallow a pill. However, devices are often mechanical, electrical and software-driven instruments, and undesired outcomes may be the result of an operator error, the wrong button being pushed or the setting being too high, or a device malfunction. Was the device dropped earlier in the day or is it a manufacturing defect? Devices may be dangerous to the operators as well as to the patients. Post-marketing safety monitoring is especially important for devices because there is often little human clinical testing of devices before they are cleared for marketing and widespread use. Most devices, about 90 %, are cleared because they are substantially equivalent to a device already on the market, and of these only about 10 % do pre-market human clinical testing. Frequent post-marketing

© Springer International Publishing Switzerland 2014
W.H. Eaglstein, *The FDA for Doctors*, DOI 10.1007/978-3-319-08362-9_20

manufacturing changes in devices also make understanding or knowing the safety of a marketed device difficult.

Drugs, by contrast, undergo extensive human pre-marketing testing during which adverse events are monitored, studied and reported to IRBs, the sponsor and FDA. Ultimately the relationship between a drug's potential benefit and risk (especially adverse events) determine its approvability by FDA. However, although not emphasized to doctors, it is important to recognize that most drugs are approved based on studies of limited numbers of subjects, in the range of 3,000, and always for relatively short periods of time. Combine these factors with the fairly restrictive criteria used for entering the studies leading to FDA approval and one quickly realizes that newly approved drugs may easily produce problems which occur rarely, or in a slightly different population than was originally studied or with prolonged usage, and that such adverse events will only be recognized after marketing. For example the biologic drug Efalizumab, known by the trade name Raptiva, was approved for the treatment of psoriasis in 2003 at which time 2,764 patients had been treated with the agent, and of them only 218 had been treated for over 1 year. Approximately 6 years later, in 2009, Efalizumab was voluntarily recalled from the market by the company because of the occurrence of progressive multifocal leuko-encephalopathy in patients taking the drug. The estimated incidence of PML, a lethal and rare disease, is estimated to be as low as one case per 2,000 users per year. Most post-marketing requirements call for reporting Serious Adverse Events. An adverse event is considered to be any undesirable experience associated with the use of a medical product in a patient. Serious adverse events that FDA requires reporting are those which cause death, threaten life, require hospitalization, produce birth defects, cause disability and events requiring surgical or medical interventions to prevent occurrences such as those mentioned. FDA also encourages reporting of medication errors especially when related to possible faulty labeling, drug names or physical identity.

The system FDA has in place for reporting and using information on adverse drug reactions is called FAERS for FDA Adverse Event Reporting System. FAERS is basically a database of information on post-marketing adverse events and medication error reports received by FDA. Reports come to FDA from doctors and other health care professionals as well as from the public, often by way of the MedWatch, which is designed for voluntary reporting by the public and health care professionals. Doctors are not usually taught in medical school or elsewhere to report adverse drug reactions occurring in the practice setting to FDA, even if they are serious. Doctors are also not likely to be looking for the opportunity to spend time filling out forms and as such they are not usually alert to the idea of reporting adverse drug events to FDA. FDA estimates that in general only about 10 % of adverse drug events and about 15 % of adverse device events are reported. Companies may also receive reports of adverse drug events and when they do they are required to report them to FDA. All of these reports are entered into the FAERS system and analysed for danger signals by FDA staff. Serious adverse events occurring with devices are required to be reported to FDA by manufacturers, importers and user facilities such as hospitals. However, often manufacturers and others may not learn of a serious adverse event until quite some time following the event when there is a lawsuit related to the event.

Overall because of the voluntary nature of most of the reporting, especially reporting by doctors, FDA's system, while useful, is often slower than those in other countries in recognizing dangers of marketed agents. Other countries also use so called registries to prospectively track devices such as heart valves and joint implants which have the potential for serious problems. FDA is thought to be considering similar approaches.

A major step toward improving drug safety, at least for drugs with the most dangerous side effects, was taken in 2007 when Congress amended the FD&C Act to authorize FDA to require risk evaluation and mitigation strategies (REMS) for especially dangerous medications (drugs and biologicals). The Act gave FDA the authority to require companies to develop REMS on any medications FDA deems to be sufficiently dangerous. The REMS may be required before a medication is marketed or, if the danger is detected after marketing, the REMS may be required in order to continue marketing. The major elements of a REMS program are a medication guide or a patient package which must be distributed to the patient with the medication, a communication plan for educating physicians and other providers, and other activities known collectively as elements to assure safe use (ETASU). These programs, while only required of the marketing company, may affect physicians in many ways, including requiring physicians to take special training and obtain certification in order to prescribe the medications, forcing physicians to enroll patients taking the medication in registry programs, or requiring physicians to issue mandatory reports of patient responses to the agents. These are extraordinary powers which indicate Congressional concern about drug safety. Among the best known drugs for which REMS are required are Thalidomide and Isotretinoin which are both able to cause birth defects.

Chapter 21
FDA Rule Making and Guidances

Although not essential to a broad understanding of FDA matters from a physician's point-of-view, how the rules governing the many areas of importance to doctors are made is in fact very important in determining how the FDA controls or is obliged to regulate much of the medical and health environment in which we practice. Developing FDA rules, even about seemingly simple matters such as, for example, the rules related to OTC sunscreens, can be a surprisingly complex activity which may take many years. FDA's intention to develop a monograph containing the rules for OTC sunscreens was first announced by FDA in 1978. A Tentative Final Monograph was published 15 years later in 1993 and the Final Monograph was published in 1999, a 21-year process. Even then the date for implementation was postponed by way of an "Extension of Effective Date", a "Partial Stay of Effective Date", a "Delay of Drug Fact Implementation", a "Technical Amendment" and a "Notice on Name Change", all of which resulted in final completion of the monograph in 2004, a 25-year long process! While this case was clearly an anomaly – most rules complete the required process within 3 years – the time needed to make FDA rules, especially when extreme as in the sunscreen monograph case, lead to considerable criticism of FDA. Rulemaking is a formal and often contentious process. And when the science or the societal views are not settled or clear, rulemaking tends to take prolonged periods of time. However, it should also be noted that in many situations during the rule making process industry tends over time to voluntarily comply with the rules they believe will ultimately apply.

Rulemaking by FDA, as with all other parts of the federal government, is a formal official process. It includes a series of required steps including publication of an Advanced Notice of Proposed Rulemaking, a Proposed Rule and a Final Rule. Importantly, there is a required Comment Period following the publication of the Proposed Rule during which any interested party may comment, object, offer alternative thinking and so forth. The publication of the Final Rule also contains a reply to all of the important comments received and must put forward the rationale and basis for the ruling. These notices and rules are all published in the Federal Register.

© Springer International Publishing Switzerland 2014
W.H. Eaglstein, *The FDA for Doctors*, DOI 10.1007/978-3-319-08362-9_21

Rules define the means or methods by which the Agency will implement laws passed by Congress and approved by the President, and carry with them the weight and force of law. When laws are passed the appropriate agency develops rules to implement the law. FDA may also create rules without a law being passed. However, all rules are legally binding, unlike the more informal Guidances which FDA may also issue. Guidances, usually entitled Guidance For Industry, are meant to outline or explain FDA's current thinking on an issue. Guidances may be published on any issues; for example, study endpoints or more technical or policy issues. One key feature of Guidances is that they are not binding on FDA or on those attempting to comply with FDA regulations. The importance of the nonbinding nature of Guidances is reflected by the statement at the top of each page of a Guidance which reads "Contains Nonbinding Recommendations" and the statement: "This guidance represents the Food and Drug Administration's (FDA's) current thinking on this topic. It does not create or confer any rights for or on any person and does not operate to bind FDA or the public. You can use an alternative approach if the approach satisfies the requirements of the applicable statutes and regulations. If you want to discuss an alternative approach, contact the FDA staff responsible for implementing this guidance. If you cannot identify the appropriate FDA staff, call the appropriate number listed on the title page of this guidance." This statement is found near the title of each Guidance in a bold black box similar to that used for key safety information on drug labels.

The process for developing Guidances is a more informal process than that required for developing rules. For example, although notice of a proposed Guidance is given and a comment period allowed, the final Guidance does not need to be changed based on the public comments received. Although the process of developing Guidances is becoming more formal, the more limited formal requirements have traditionally allowed Guidances to be produced more quickly than Rules, and made Guidances more useful for situations in which the science underlying them is uncertain or evolving rapidly. Partially for these reasons FDA issues about three times more Guidances than Rules. Overall, Guidances have been well received by industry which not only appreciates the instructions but is very keen for the relative certainty and consistency Guidances offer to the development and regulatory process as well as to the competitive market place.

Chapter 22
Enforcement and Warning Letters

The FDA reports its enforcement activities in the following categories: seizures (taking possession of a product to keep it off of the market), injunctions (to stop an action which violates a law), warning letters, recalls, and debarments (Table 22.1).

Injunctions against companies, seizure of products and recall of products are all vigorous actions which are often in response to immediate safety concerns and which are usually given wide press coverage, especially when the public needs to be warned of dangers from foods, drugs or other regulated products. Warning letters are not as widely publicized but are highly reflective of FDA's approach to problems and its endeavor to elicit voluntary compliance. Until FDA's recent activities related to tobacco sales, the number of warning letters ranged from 400 to 700 annually. Warning letters are not required to be sent before FDA takes an action but when possible are a preferred approach, aimed at obtaining voluntary cooperation. Warning letters notify the firm or responsible person that FDA considers one or more of its activities, practices, processes or products to be in violation of the FD&C Act or one of the regulations based on the Act or other federal regulation.

In addition to spelling out the observed or detected violations the letter contains specific instruction as to what a firm is expected to do in response to the letter. The response, usually required within 15 days, is to include a written description of each step that has been or will be taken to correct the violations and prevent them in the future; the time in which the correction will be finished; reasons the action has not been taken or done in the time expected; and the documentation to show the correction has been made. Corrective actions may be quite significant, such as withdrawal of a product from the market, in this case a voluntary withdrawal. Other corrective actions of great interest to doctors may be the withdrawal of a drug advertisement or other promotion and issuance of a correction. Although FDA does not send letters unless the violation is considered significant, FDA does not have to take action and will not if the response is satisfactory. However, Warning Letters are posted on FDA's websites and even if there is no further action the letters may cause unexpected problems for the company and its management team.

© Springer International Publishing Switzerland 2014
W.H. Eaglstein, *The FDA for Doctors*, DOI 10.1007/978-3-319-08362-9_22

Table 22.1 FDA
enforcement – 2013 summary

Type of action	Number
Seizures	6
Injunctions	19
Warning letters	6,760
Recall events	3,844
Recalled products	8,044
Debarments	6

FDA enforcement activities fall into a number of categories. Until FDA's recent tobacco sales enforcement activities the number of warning letters was in the 400–700/year range

Debarments refer to FDA action against individuals, including its own employees, or companies who engage in criminal conduct with respect to the development or approval of new drugs. The debarment authority was granted in a 1992 law and prohibits the person or company from participating in any activity leading to submission of a new drug application. Debarment is mostly applied to individuals, usually after they have been found guilty by a court, although that is not needed, and effectively prevents them from working in the drug industry. Courts have upheld this penalty as needed to protect the public.

The FDA, which regulates and carries out both announced and unannounced inspections/audits of clinical trials (clinical investigative sites) used for regulatory approval, has the authority to disqualify clinical investigators either permanently or temporarily from participating in clinical trials leading to FDA approval and from receiving investigational materials and devices via interstate commerce. Clinical investigators who conduct these studies are required to comply with applicable statutes and regulations intended to ensure the integrity of clinical data upon which product approvals are based and for research involving human subjects, to help protect the rights, safety, and welfare of those subjects. When FDA alleges a clinical investigator has violated applicable regulations, FDA may initiate a clinical investigator disqualification proceeding. These are FDA administrative proceedings (not a court activity) and offer the doctor or other qualified clinical investigator the opportunity to explain why regulations were not followed. FDA may accept the explanation, but if not the investigator may be disqualified. FDA websites provide a list of disqualified clinical investigators often including a description of the basis for the disqualification and information from the hearing.

Chapter 23
The FDA, Politics and Criticism

An organization charged with regulating nearly 25 % of the country's economy, including the food supply, human and veterinary medicines, tobacco and cosmetics, not only cannot remain free from criticism but must by necessity be perceived as unfair and performing poorly by one or another of the many elements of society affected by its activities. Focusing only on the biomedical industry, FDA- regulated activities employ an estimated 1.5 million people plus over 6 million people in its supply chain, all of whom are likely at one time or another to be directly impacted by an FDA decision.

On the macro political scale, since FDA is under the jurisdiction of the Department of Health and Human Services whose head is appointed by the President as is the head of the FDA itself, the potential for not only real politically-oriented intervention and policy making but also for the perception of such is great. For example, the unusual decision by the HHS Secretary Kathleen Sebelius in 2011 to overrule FDA's approval of the Plan B contraceptive pill being sold from the aisle, which would allow teenage girls to buy it without a prescription or assistance, was widely criticized and perceived by some to be a move by President Obama to appease conservatives, and was an unusually highly visible "political" decision.

While few regulatory decisions are made with input at such high levels by presidential appointees, almost all FDA decisions singly and in aggregate are perceived by someone to be good or bad and often political. FDA is in reality in a "no win" situation most of the time. For example, to those wanting access to as yet unapproved or unproven drugs FDA is too conservative, leading to people suffering or dying because of excess regulatory caution. This is especially true when a drug or agent is approved in other countries but not the U.S. When people suffer serious drug side effects, especially those not recognized upon initial approval and labeling, FDA is often considered to be at fault for insufficient concern and for being more interested in fostering drug company profit by easy and hurried approvals than in public safety. Issues of over-regulation and under-regulation are mainstays of FDA criticism and are often played out with a political twist.

© Springer International Publishing Switzerland 2014
W.H. Eaglstein, *The FDA for Doctors*, DOI 10.1007/978-3-319-08362-9_23

A powerful assertion is that FDA is biased toward non-approval of agents because the damage done to people failing to receive the benefits of a new treatment is less visible than the damage done to people when an approved agent causes harm. For doctors this is similar to our famous admonition to "do no harm", but not having an explicit injunction that tells us "do not fail to do good". Indeed one of FDA's most highly revered actions was its refusal to approved Thalidomide, thus sparing the United States' public the disastrous birth defects induced by Thalidomide. Ironically this refusal to approve, which was based on a safety concern (thyroid function) and avoided approval of a drug unsafe for pregnant women, led to the law requiring that in addition to being safe, drugs must be proven effective before they could be marketed. Even this requirement, that before approval drugs must be proven to work, has been criticized as leading to a slower and more expensive approval process which has done more harm than good and cost more lives than it has saved. This criticism is often combined with the observation that prior to the 1962 efficacy requirement, drugs were approved in about 7 months, but some 30 years later development time averaged over 7 years. As noted elsewhere, FDA was very effectively pressured by the AIDS community about its policies which limited access to unapproved treatments and about its slow approval process. Ultimately FDA's processes for faster drug approvals led to many anti AIDS drugs being first approved in the United States.

With User Fees, which are paid to FDA by industry, now accounting for nearly half of FDA's annual operating budget, the charge that industry has captured its regulators is perhaps more plausible than ever before. Books are written and even films are made about the evil industrial elements' unending quest for profits at the expense of public health. Even the failure to approve drugs made by foreign companies that are approved elsewhere is seen by some critics as FDA protecting domestic industry. A similar situation is seen in the food regulatory arena. FDA's allowance of certain food additives, including certain coloring agents, antibiotics and hormones to speed growth and increase milk production in healthy animals, certain fertilizers and food processing techniques, all of which are thought by critics to be harmful to humans, is perceived to be the result of the food industry having "captured" the regulatory agency. In addition to such policy-based issues, FDA is constantly subject to criticism based on its operations and application of policies. For example, the time needed to get a meeting with FDA staff in order to clarify an issue for a development program may be some months, during which development will be slowed. Another frequent complaint relates to FDA changing its approval requirements after an agreement with the sponsor has been reached and the development has been completed based on the agreement. This sort of so-called last minute change is often consequent upon new information becoming available to FDA since the original agreement. This might seem inevitable given the long time needed to implement and complete many of the studies needed as part of the approval package.

Returning to the more overtly political, it should be kept in mind, that Congress can still make or change laws which dictate FDA activities. The special laws passed by congress dictating that supplements should be regulated as foods rather than drugs, but allowing certain classes of health claims, is a good example. When people, organizations, companies and industries feel imposed upon or wish to simply change their circumstances vis-a-vis the FDA, they and their lobbyists contact their federal senators and congressmen. These legislators have access to FDA's legislative affairs offices and others in the agency and in HHS who are able to transmit their constituents' concerns and on occasion effect changes. FDA's importance is reflected in the many articles and editorials in the press and in magazines and in the host of publications focusing exclusively on FDA activities.

The centrality of FDA's role in our society, which almost by definition will be seen as having a political element, is very well-illustrated in its recent attempts to lead us in dealing with the creation of humans by three-person fertilization. FDA's recent 2-day meeting about a new in vitro fertilization technique which would use the DNA of three people (mother, father and mitochondrial donor) places FDA in the center of key social issues, such as the creation of "designer" children. For many people facilitation or precluding such activity will be viewed as political. From designer children to deciding whether the information technology systems used in health care should be regulated for safety as are other "medical" devices, FDA's role remains so broad as to be constantly bound up in the "political".

Chapter 24
Brief History of the FDA

This book is intended to inform doctors about today's FDA and yet, as with a patient's disease state or current health, the history contributes enormously to our understanding of the current status. With that in mind, a brief history of the FDA including some of the major lessons from that history will help in understanding the current organization and its outlook and biases. Broadly speaking, FDA was created and exists today because of commercial abuse and misbehavior, especially as regards food processing, food additives and patent medicines. Many, if not most, of the major revisions of FDA's role, including expansions of its authority, have been in response to various public health disasters and the desire to prevent recurrences or similar problems.

Doctors might be pleased to learn that the legislation leading ultimately to creation of the FDA was in great measure the result of work by a person trained in medicine. The passage by Congress in 1906 of the Pure Food and Drugs Act, also known at the time as the Wiley Act, is generally considered to have come about because of the efforts of Dr. Harvey W. Wiley, who is widely known as the "Father of the FDA". Histories of this era also credit the exposure of unsanitary conditions in the meat industry, especially in the popular book *The Jungle* by Upton Sinclair, with helping to develop the broad-based societal support needed to allow passage of the new law. The 1906 act prohibited entering adulterated or misbranded food and drugs into interstate commerce. The 1906 act did not explicitly require that drugs be either safe or effective.

Dr. Wiley, who was also trained and worked primarily as a chemist analyzing agricultural products, worked for some time as Chief Chemist of the Bureau of Chemistry in the Department of Agriculture. In this capacity he also conducted studies in which healthy individuals ate contaminated foods in order to study their effects. These investigative human studies were done on a group of human volunteers formed by Wiley in 1902 which became famously known as the "poison squad". Among other things, they studied the effects on digestion and health of various food preservatives, coloring matters and other substances used, often inappropriately, in foods and patent medicines of the era. This work helped expose abuses

W.H. Eaglstein, *The FDA for Doctors*, DOI 10.1007/978-3-319-08362-9_24

and unsafe material in processed foods and patent medicines. Dr. Wiley lobbied for the creation of food and drug legislation for over 25 years before its ultimate passage. Clearly, the time lines of the present are not so different than those of the past.

The 1906 Act added regulatory functions to the Bureau's scientific activity and in 1927 the Bureau of Chemistry's name changed to the Food, Drug and Insecticide Administration. Three years later the name was amended to the Food and Drug Administration. Although a great step forward, the regulatory authority given in the 1906 Act rested on the ability to demand products not be adulterated or mislabeled/ misbranded. However, medicines, because they needn't prove safety prior to marketing, could avoid the charge of mislabeling by not suggesting what uses a medicine might have. This strategy allowed many unsafe drug products to be marketed. It was not until over 100 people died from what was called a Sulfanilamide Elixir but which in fact was Sulfanilamide dissolved in the toxic solvent diethylene glycol rather than ethanol, that legislation was passed in 1938 which gave FDA authority to require pre-market review of drug safety.

The so called Sulfanilamide Elixir disaster is not well known by doctors today but it is very informative and illustrative even today. The drug sulfanilamide, dispensed as a powder or a tablet had been found to be curative for streptococcal infections. In June 1937 however, a salesman for the S.E. Massengill Co. in Bristol, TN reported a demand in the southern states for the drug in liquid form. The company's chief chemist and pharmacist experimented and found that sulfanilamide would dissolve in diethylene glycol. Company tests for appearance, fragrance and flavor were satisfactory and within months the company sent it for use throughout the country. Since it was a known active pharmaceutical agent (drug), toxicity testing and pharmacology studies were not done, so the fact that the vehicle, which was used primarily as an antifreeze, was highly toxic was not determined by the company. Within a few months the deadly nature of the "elixir" was recognized but chasing down and recovering the already distributed drug required a great deal of time and utilized all of the 239 FDA inspectors and chemists. About 234 gallons of the 240 gallons produced were eventually recovered. Over 100 people in 15 states from Virginia to California had died.

Because FDA had only authority over misbranding, if the drug had been labeled a solution rather than a tincture FDA would not have had the legal right to recover/ recall the drug from the market because it would not have been mislabeled. The new formulation had not been tested for toxicity. At the time the food and drugs law did not require that safety studies be done on new drugs. Selling toxic drugs was, undoubtedly, bad for business and could damage a firm's reputation, but it was not illegal. Although the company insisted it had not acted illegally, the chemist inventor committed suicide over the incident and as noted this disaster also led to major legislation.

This new law, passed in 1938 largely in response to the Sulfanilamide disaster and known as The Federal Food, Drug and Cosmetic Act of 1938 or simply the Food Drug and Cosmetic Act (FD&C Act), was another step along the path toward our present circumstance. In addition to requiring, for the first time, that new drugs be safe before marketing, the FD&C Act also gave FDA the power to inspect factories, provided more standards for food safety, and brought cosmetics and devices under the agency's authority. It is still the fundamental law underpinning FDA's authority.

Perhaps surprisingly it was not until 1951 that prescription drugs were defined and brought under FDA (Federal) control. Doctors of today may not realize that prior to the 1951 Durham-Murphy Amendment if a manufacturer, pharmacist or physician felt a drug should be sold only by prescription they labeled it "to be dispensed by prescription". Otherwise it was assumed the drug was over-the –counter and had to have adequate direction for use on the label. This 1951 Act also set conditions on the number of times and how a drug might be refilled, a right held dear by pharmacists of the time. As we see is often true, the case of a disastrous under treatment of a disease (gonorrhea) by OTC self- treatment in military base towns, ultimately led to this amendment allowing FDA to define which drugs were to be prescription drugs taken under the directions of a doctor.

Although FDA had been trying to force companies to assure efficacy by analyzing the amount of active agent in critical drugs and forcing agents which seem to be ineffective off the market by designating them as mislabeled, it was not until passage in 1962 of the Kefauver-Harris Amendment to the FD&C Act that pre-market proof of efficacy was a clear requirement. The Kefauver-Harris Amendment contained a number of major reforms and was a bill which, again, was passed primarily in response to a public health disaster. However on this occasion the disaster, the induction of birth defects by the drug Thalidomide given to combat morning sickness in pregnancy, occurred in Europe but not the United States. Thalidomide was not approved for marketing in the United States because of the efforts of Francis Kelsey, Ph.D., M.D., an FDA reviewer, who was concerned about Thalidomide's potential to cause thyroid toxicity. Because she prevented approval, Dr. Kelsey is one of FDA's public health heroes and was awarded the highest civilian award of the Federal Government. FDA critics often note that Kelsey's heroic act was to prevent a drug from reaching the market rather than to have helped assure speedy availability of a drug to market.

During the nearly 25 years since passage of the 1938 FD&C Act requiring pre-market safety, over 3,400 drugs for over 16,000 indications had been approved for marketing based only on their being considered safe. The Kefauver-Harris Amendment required that those drugs be evaluated and if not found to be effective, to be withdrawn from the market. To evaluate the efficacy of all of the drugs approved and marketed before 1962, FDA developed a process called the Drug Efficacy Study Implementation, hence the name DESI. This was a large undertaking which because of limited resources FDA contracted to the National Academy of Sciences/National Research Council and in which many doctors throughout the country participated on a basically volunteer basis. The review process was not started until many years after the pre-market safety requirement was passed, and while never fully completed the process was discontinued in 1984, by which time the available studies and literature had been reviewed and conclusions and rulings had been made with most (2,225) of the 3,400 pre-1962 drugs ruled to be effective and allowed to stay on the market. Others were withdrawn or went through a new but abbreviated approval process while some were never adjudicated and remain on the market today as so called DESI drugs. (See Chap. 2).

In considerable measure because of the Kefauver Amendment requirement that market approval be contingent upon demonstrating "substantial evidence" of effectiveness, by the 1970s the United States faced what became known as the "drug lag". While not a public health disaster, the drug lag was a situation in which many new drugs were first approved for marketing in other countries. These new drugs were not available to patients in the United States and companies were "deprived" of the revenues from the United States. Because the pre-market efficacy requirement necessitated studies that prolonged the development process, the amount of patent protected marketing time available after approval was reduced. This in turn reduced the incentive to develop new drugs. In response to many of the pressures occasioned by the loss of useful patent time and the drug lag, the Drug Price Competition and Patent Term Restoration Act, more commonly known as the "Hatch-Waxman Act" was enacted in 1984. This act, as suggested in its name, restored or extended the patent time to somewhat compensate for the time lost in complying with the FDA's pre-market approval requirements (See Chap. 10). In addition, the Hatch-Waxman Act created the Abbreviated New Drug Application mechanism, which encouraged the development of generic drugs in part by allowing generic drugs to be approved based on surrogate endpoints, such as drug blood levels, rather than the costly process of treating people with diseases in clinical trials. Many credit Waxman-Hatch with not only generating a real generic drug industry in the United States but also by way of the patent restoration portion of the act have either moved us to the forefront for drug development again or kept us there.

The public health disaster known as the AIDS epidemic was the motor behind a significant group of revolutionary changes in the agency's regulations regarding compassionate use of experimental drugs, and approval of drugs for life threatening diseases without alternative treatments. Although cancer sufferers and those suffering a number of other untreatable, lethal and life destroying diseases had the same needs, the AIDS patients, by virtue of being fairly young and early in their disease, still vigorous and quickly able to develop a large, informed and highly connected community, were able to bring a greater and more effective level of political pressure on the FDA than people suffering other diseases. In response to the public protests and political pressure, FDA altered or made new regulations which resulted in rapid approvals of new anti-AIDS drugs, reduced the difficulty of importing unapproved drugs for personal use and improved access to unapproved investigational drugs. These policies have not only helped with the development of treatments and diagnostics for AIDS but also for other lethal and serious diseases.

Finally as noted elsewhere, the high levels of avoidable disease caused by or associated with smoking, which some perceived to be a public health crisis if not a disaster, led to actions by the federal government such as the declaration by the surgeon general that cigarettes cause lung cancer and FDA's assertion of authority over tobacco advertising to youngsters. Ultimately, following challenges to its authority over tobacco advertising and other FDA tobacco rules, Congress passed the Family Smoking Prevention and Tobacco Control Act in 2009. This act authorized FDA to regulate the manufacture, marketing and distribution of tobacco products to protect public health and to reduce tobacco use. It did not allow FDA to ban the sale of tobacco products thereby putting FDA in the position of regulating a product which is considered to be unhealthy and unsafe.

As I hope is clear from this brief history, most of the major changes in the laws or the regulations related to FDA's authority and jurisdiction are the result of a real and publicly recognized public health problem, usually characterized as disastrous. Upon reflection, considering that almost any change in how the products within FDA's jurisdiction are regulated, or that the placement of unregulated products into FDA's regulatory orbit will directly or indirectly harm or benefit many parties, it is not surprising that significant change can only be agreed to when there is a tremendous political will and a popular desire for the change, which are usually only present after a disaster.

Index

© Springer International Publishing Switzerland 2014   95
W.H. Eaglstein, *The FDA for Doctors*, DOI 10.1007/978-3-319-08362-9